stress management

in essence

Jennie Harding

Series Editor: Nicola Jenkins

Hodder Arnold

A MEMBER OF THE HODDER HEADLINE GROUP

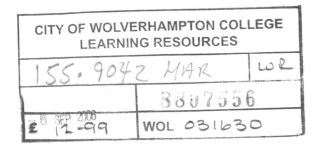
Orders: please contact Bookpoint Ltd, 130 Milton Park, Abingdon, Oxon OX14 4SB. Telephone: (44) 01235 827720. Fax: (44) 01235 400454. Lines are open from 9.00 – 5.00, Monday to Saturday, with a 24 hour message answering service. You can also order through our website www.hoddereducation.co.uk

If you have any comments to make about this, or any of our other titles, please send them to educationenquiries@hodder.co.uk

British Library Cataloguing in Publication Data
A catalogue record for this title is available from the British Library

ISBN-10: 0 340 92607 4
ISBN-13: 978 0 340 92607 9

First Edition Published 2006
Impression number   10 9 8 7 6 5 4 3 2 1
Year   2011 2010 2009 2008 2007 2006

Hodder Headline's policy is to use papers that are natural, renewable and recyclable products and made from wood grown in sustainable forests. The logging and manufacturing processes are expected to conform to the environmental regulations of the country of origin.

Cover photo by Chris Cole/Photographer's Choice/Getty Images

Typeset by Servis Filmsetting Ltd, Manchester
Printed in Great Britain for Hodder Arnold, an imprint of Hodder Education, a member of the Hodder Headline Group, 338 Euston Road, London NW1 3BH, by CPI Bath.

acknowledgements

My thanks to my dear friends Ann and Ray Burger for allowing me to write in the peace and quiet of their home. This book is dedicated to them.

The author and publishers would like to thank the following for the use of photographs in this volume.

p. 3 Alan Marler/AP © Empics, p. 5 Mary Evans Picture Library, pp. 6–9, 24–26, 29, 36, 46, 59, 69, 70 (left), 100–101 Ingrams, pp. 14, 67–8, 70 (right), 71, 88, 95, 99 Photodisc, p. 17 Art Kowalsky/Alamy, p. 19 LWA-Stephen Welstead © Corbis, p. 26 Image Source/Alamy, p. 48 © Royalty-Free/Corbis, p. 49 John Arnold Images © Photolibrary, p. 50 Botanica/Photolibrary, p. 58 Photononstop/Photolibrary, p. 60 Mary Evans Picture Library, p. 62 Workbook, Inc © Photolibrary, p. 63 Foodpix © Photolibrary, p. 72 © Royalty-Free/Corbis, p. 80 Plainpicture © Photolibrary, p. 81 Index Stock Imagery © Photolibrary, p. 82 Aflo Foto Agency © Photolibrary, p. 83 Stock 4b Gmbh © Photolibrary, p. 96 Mauritius Die Bildagentur Gmbh © Photolibrary, p. 98 Photolibrary.com (Australia).

Commissioned photographs by Carl Drury.

contents

introduction

Welcome to *Stress Management in Essence,* and the beginning of a wonderful journey. That idea might surprise you, given that this book is going to be about stress. For most of us, that word conjures up pictures of discomfort and pain, trials and tribulations or setbacks and problems. What we are going to explore is the fact that life events are often made worse by stress, so by unlocking and understanding what stress is we can start to understand it and deal with things much more positively. This does not have to be a painful process either; in fact, it can shed light on all aspects of our lives and give us new tools to help ourselves.

This book is a practical manual that will guide you to a much wider understanding of what stress is, how it works and how it can affect your life. Reading and working with the ideas shown here will demonstrate that dealing with stress can be really informative and even a fun thing to do. The word 'stress' is bandied about so much these days, but do we really know what it is? Well, after this journey you will have a much better idea.

If you can bring an open mind, a sense of humour and a dose of honest self-observation to this journey, you will really reap the benefits. This book is not intended as a course of personal therapy, nor is it designed to train you as a stress-management counsellor. Later on you will find out how to take your understanding of stress management further if you want to, but the aim of this book is to stimulate ideas and thoughts at a simple level that is easy to understand. We will do that by asking you to take a look at different aspects of yourself and how you react to situations, purely to enable you to make this journey your own. A little practice goes a long way and makes a theory feel real. However, it is also important to stress that you don't have to lay your inner self open to anyone here; if you are using this book as part of a course, then your tutor will guide you as to what is appropriate for you to share in the classroom situation. You always have the final choice as to what feels right for you. Again, the aim of this journey is to stimulate ideas and not to put you through a course of therapeutic treatment.

Having said that, if by exploring some of the aspects of this journey you do feel issues are highlighted for you that need further guidance and personal exploration, then there are many branches of professional therapy that can help you. At the end of the book we will look at some of these so that you can consider your choices.

Why study stress at all? Well, perhaps because it is a fact of modern life and it affects us all at some time or other, but it's also something that is very personal: it touches each one of us in a different way. It is very easy to go through life on a treadmill, burdened more and more by the build-up of stress, experiencing its effects and feeling powerless to do anything about them. However, we don't need to be at its mercy and we really can help ourselves. If we are willing to take a clear and honest look at our lives and apply some simple principles, then things can really start to change.

Change is really at the heart of the picture, and it is a fact of existence that is beyond doubt these days. Whether you consider the environment, work, economics, geography, family life or the weather, recent world events are showing that change is at work on a scale that is vast and multifaceted. For example, only one generation ago, expectations of a 'job for life' were common and people felt they could project an idea of how their life might be over decades. Now it is barely possible to project a year ahead – and perhaps not even that far. People are being hit by waves of change that can seem overwhelming and, again, a sense of powerlessness can bring deep levels of emotional stress. However, change is also exciting and empowering if you can turn your perceptions around. Later in this book

we will look at some ways of starting to do this for yourself.

Although this book is designed as a progression of ideas, each of the ten chapters is self-contained and within each one you will find different kinds of material. For example, there will be quizzes and exercises that you are invited to use to think about things that affect you, either on your own or in the classroom. We will be looking at some case study examples of different situations to highlight strategies for dealing with them. You will find frequently asked questions (FAQs) at the end of each chapter to highlight typical issues. It's a really good idea to start writing in a special notebook as you work through the chapters, whether you are using this book to support a stress-management course in adult education or using it on your own. This will allow you to keep all your jottings, answers to quizzes, thoughts, questions and other notes in one place. It also makes a kind of diary as you go through the ten chapters and you may very well find at the end that going back over your notes gives you a tremendous sense of how far you have come on your journey.

In the end, this journey is about YOU. It allows you to think about things such as, Why do I act like this? How do I want to be seen? How do I want to live my life? Do I want to be a puppet on strings pulled by stress, or do I want to take a good look at myself and find out how I can make things better? You decide, you choose. You may be surprised at how much fun you have while you find out.

the nature
of stress

In the first three chapters we will be looking at ways to understand what stress is and how it affects us all. You will be encouraged to think about areas in your life where stress has an impact on you. This foundation will prepare you to learn the methods of dealing with stress later in the book.

exploring stress

'Stress' is a word that can mean many things. If you are speaking, it can mean that you put emphasis on a particular thing you say to stress your point. If you are a scientist, you could use the word to mean putting pressure on an object until it shows a breaking point. If you are a fitness expert, you could say that extreme activity places stress on muscles to the point of them failing. If you are climbing a mountain, slip, and are left hanging on a rope over a cliff edge, those combined circumstances could be said to place you under extreme emotional stress through fear.

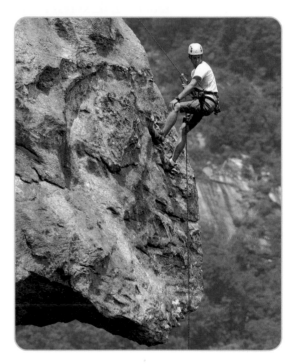

Hanging off a cliff can be a stressful situation unless you have the tools to cope with it

3

The root of the word 'stress' comes from Old French, the language of the Norman Conquest which took place nearly 1,000 years ago, where *estresse* meant narrowness, straightness or oppression. It is interesting to look at this – the most ancient meaning of the word already implies a force that is pressing or squeezing things into tightness or constriction. How does that compare with the way you feel when you think about the effects you associate normally with stress?

In this chapter we are going to explore what your concepts of stress are at the moment, to see how you think about it and express it and how you think it affects your life. We will look at a case study exercise to highlight certain aspects of stress; you will also have the chance to think about some of your own experiences of stress and how they seem to affect you. This chapter will pave the route for the journey to follow by allowing you to set down some ideas of your own before we get into more depth as far as study is concerned. This is important because throughout the rest of the book, we are encouraging you to observe, to think and to consider how the material relates to you. That is why these exercises are needed – and they are fun to do!

What do you think stress is?

Take a few moments, either in your group or on your own, to make a list of the words you associate most closely with 'stress'. This works best if you just write what comes straight into your head. Then compare notes with your classmates, see what they came up with, or examine your list to see if there are any trends, any themes, which come up again and again.

A prominent theme is likely to be pressure. Stress often feels like something that crushes you, something that presses down on you and makes you feel helpless.

Perhaps some of you highlighted emotions, like fear, anxiety, worry; or the effects of stress like feeling breathless, your heart racing or your palms becoming damp. All these things help to build up a picture of what stress might look like – and already you can see it is complex. It is not easy to narrow it down. Sometimes it seems to link to emotions, sometimes to effects, sometimes to things from outside you and sometimes to things inside you. In fact, stress is all these things and more – a truly compact idea with many facets.

How modern is humankind?

Here is an exercise that has some interesting things to show you about human stress and how it operates. It is based on actual elements of human physiology, which are relatively unchanged after a million or so years of evolution. There are two scenarios to examine individually and then compare. You will find questions to guide you at the end of each one.

casestudy

Scenario 1 – Prehistoric man

Imagine a prehistoric man walking vast plains in search of animals to hunt for food. Here he is in a very wide open space, and he has to use all his senses – sight, hearing, taste, touch and smell – to find the trail of the animals he is looking for. He is walking along carefully and he is alert, primed to pick up any signs, his heart rate is up slightly and there is a tingle of blood in his limbs, a feeling that at any point he may have to run. However, this is a comfortable state for him, he is poised and ready. Then all of a sudden there is an unexpected rustling in the bushes and something unknown is coming towards him; he smells a big animal and hears its growl. All the blood rushes from his stomach and vital organs to his arms and legs and in seconds he is running for his life, his heart pumping, his lungs expanding and deflating rapidly, his muscles expanding and contracting to

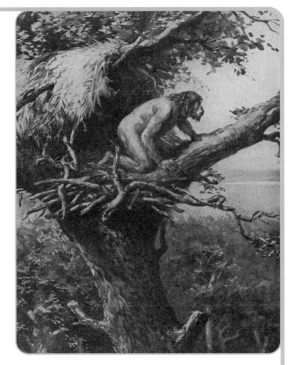

Ancient man wandered over a vast landscape and needed to stay alert

power him forward. He sees a tree ahead and dives up onto the lowest branch, quickly climbing as far as he can go, knowing the creature can't get at him. His heart continues to pound, he is sweating, his mouth is dry. The creature stays around for a while then retreats, losing interest. After some time, the man's breathing slows down, his temperature regularises itself, and he feels exhaustion in his muscles. He will rest, perhaps even sleep, until he feels strong enough to go on.

Consider these questions

1 Can you identify the pattern of activity here in the story? Look at how he starts out, then at the changes that happen.

2 If that pattern were a curve, could you draw it?

3 What is the emotion that prompted his reaction to run?

4 Do you think this had a positive or a negative effect on him?

casestudy

Scenario 2 – City man

Here is a typical city man on the move with a briefcase, laptop computer and mobile phone. Although he is walking the streets he is actually talking to someone a long way away from where he is and therefore his actual focus is not on his immediate surroundings, he maintains enough awareness just to know where he's walking. This conversation is not going well, the person he's talking to has a problem and he's a long way from fixing it but he feels under pressure. He's frowning as he walks and talks, he feels irritated, he's sweating a little under the arms. His heart rate is also up slightly but he doesn't notice. He comes off the phone and it rings again, this time it's his wife, there is a problem with one of their children. He feels pushed and is not very receptive to her need for support, he is short with her. He feels bad about that when he comes off the phone, and steps out into the street without thinking. A car nearly runs into him, it screeches to a stop and he's lucky it misses him. The driver shouts at him. It's a shock and suddenly his heart is racing, he even feels as though he has slight chest pains. He stops on the side of the road out of breath and even feels slightly giddy. He has to lean against a lamp-post until he feels better and can go on.

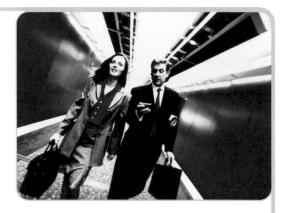

Modern man spends a lot of time doing many things at once

Consider these questions

1 As before, can you describe the pattern of the response in this man from the start of the story onwards?

2 If you could draw a curve of this story, how would it look?

3 What kind of feelings or emotions are affecting him?

4 What physical effects are happening to him?

Now let's take a look at these two scenarios and compare them. First, let's see if we can find some parallels between them, things they both have in common. Here are one or two ideas to get you started:

- In both stories the man was doing something else when the main stress event happened.

- In both stories the man experienced a strong emotional reaction to an outside event that had a physical effect on him.

- In both stories the man rested after the stressful event.

See if you can find any other similarities between the stories.

Then let's contrast the two accounts and see how they are different to each other. Think about how they show the varied reactions of the two men. Again, here are one or two points to get you started.

- In the first, the man is alert but comfortable at the beginning. In the second, he's under pressure from the start.
- In the first, the man is very aware of his environment. In the second, the man is somewhere else in his head.
- In the first, the man only gets into a really stressed state when he senses the creature nearby. In the second, the man is constantly under pressure from one thing or another.

Again, think about the contrasts carefully and note as many as you can.

The point about both of these scenarios is that they are in fact very similar in terms of what is happening to the human body. When it comes to our physical selves we are still very like the prehistoric man who has a strong survival mechanism that kicks in when he is in danger. As we will see in the next chapter, this is called the 'fight or flight' response. It allows a massive amount of energy to be released to give us the best chance of getting out of danger and recovering afterwards, as happened when the prehistoric man had to run for his life as a result of fear. However, in the case of the city man, he has the same kind of body and the same ability to react, but his life is made up of a much more complicated set of events, which he is trying to deal with all at once – work problems, family issues, etc. – using the technology which modern society has developed. You could ask yourself whether

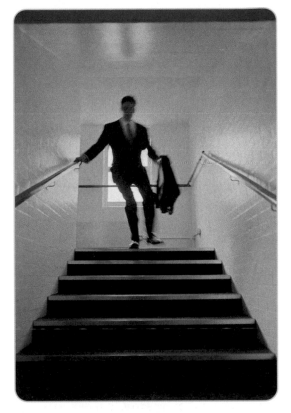

The 'fight-or-flight' mechanism sends a lot of energy to the muscles

that technology is really helping him or, rather, contributing to his stress levels. However, what is also key with him is that he is experiencing lots of anxiety peaks, one after another – through fear, worry about performance, irritation at things he can't deal with – and these culminate in his loss of survival awareness, so he nearly gets run over and his heart is working so hard he develops chest pains. There has been no time for him to recover from any of these peaks so they are building up in intensity. It is no surprise, therefore, that increasingly stressful life events can be strong factors in heart attacks, one of the biggest killers of our time. This is because we have an ancient physiology that does not always adapt very easily to the constant levels of stress in modern life. However, the good news is it can be helped and, in the chapters ahead, we will start to find out how.

Another important thing to notice at this point is that our human inbuilt stress response is designed to help and protect us. It's there to get us to a peak of physical possibility where we can do things a little beyond our ordinary efforts. This can have profound consequences for us: maybe by being tested we actually learn something new. For instance, our prehistoric man gets out of a potentially life-threatening situation by running and using his wits in a heightened state to figure out how to survive. The energy released by that special response can be transforming – yet it is stimulated by stress. In limited amounts, this kind of

response can have some positive effects; if the body and mind experience too much of it then the situation can lead to overload.

After all this exertion the physical body needs to rest. How simple that sounds – we need to relax, to recover from the events we have experienced. Our prehistoric man does that easily in his environment and he may even stay where he is until he feels strong enough to go on. Our city man might have more of a problem with this. Do you think he ever really rests properly? He could well be the type of man who takes work home and never wholly switches off. He would probably say that he doesn't have time to do nothing. However, as we shall see through the chapters of this book, learning different ways to relax is a vital element in effective stress management.

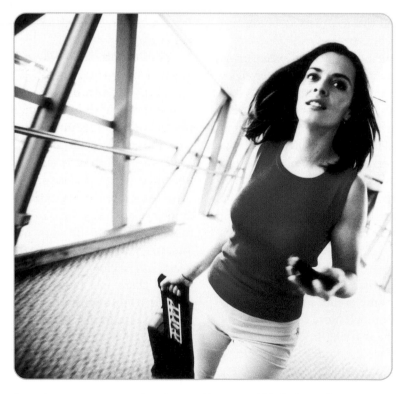

Sometimes stress can push us in a positive way which feels good

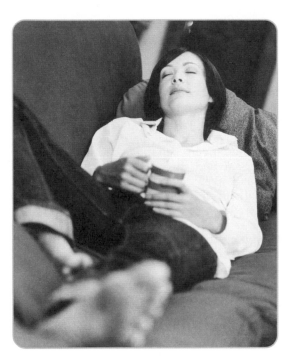

Resting after exertion allows the body to repair itself

equally balanced in your life or are some more demanding than others? Which is most dominant? If you were to draw a pie chart divided into these three areas, how would the three sections look? Would one be bigger than all the others? Try it now. If you don't have all three sections, then that is very interesting . . . the missing one may well be rather significant.

This brings up a very important point for all the exercises and tasks still to come. What you write down is personal to you and you don't have to share it if you don't want to. Also if you can be honest about yourself that is really helpful, and the notes or results you see on the page are not there to make you criticise yourself. They are simply there to be observed. We have a long way to go yet, and there will be lots of tools coming up to help you make useful changes as you see fit. Keeping notes helps you to have material to refer back to and will prove useful later on.

This chapter has allowed you to explore more closely what you think stress is and how it occurs in the moment. You have seen some important physiological effects it can have on both body and mind. You have also identified a few key areas in your life in terms of their overall importance and significance. In Chapter 2 we will explore the physiological effects of stress in more detail.

Though our two scenarios are just exercises, they contain many threads that may be familiar to you. In modern times, life can feel like a balancing act and the pressure to perform becomes intolerable. How is the balance between activity and rest in *your* life? Take three areas – work, personal relationships and relaxation. Sit quietly and think about yourself. Are these three areas

9

FAQs

When I get very stressed I feel my stomach tighten and when my friend here does, she feels she can't talk because her throat gets choked. Why are we different?

We all react to stress in a variety of ways, and often these are linked to emotions and feelings. Later on we will look at some ways of identifying the underlying feelings and how to deal with them. Basically, everyone has their own pattern, but it's great that you are already identifying these signs.

I've read that if we had no stress we would just be like blobs sitting around with no reactions at all.

This is true, and it comes back to the idea that we need some simulation to get the best out of ourselves. However, too much is not helpful and we have to get that balance right.

How can you compare a prehistoric man to a modern man when life is so different now?

I'm not comparing their lifestyles which, of course, are totally different. The case studies reflect completely different kinds of society, but what I am looking at is the fact that the human body and human physiology have changed very little over millennia. Even separated by time, the emotional and physical reactions of our two examples to stressful situations are similar. So, our lifestyle has changed but how we react to stress has not.

Do you mean that the prehistoric man is better at coping with stress than the modern man?

No, but what happens there is a single highly stressful situation, which he deals with and then recovers from. The modern man is unaware of what is happening to him, keeps on pushing himself repeatedly and is therefore more at risk from potential physiological failure.

Can being pushed beyond your limits be good for you?

Yes, in certain circumstances. Some situations, challenging as they may appear at first, can bring out the best in people by taking them to a new level of awareness about themselves and their capabilities. The knack is to keep balanced by knowing how to help yourself recover afterwards. Too much stimulation can lead to overload.

I haven't got all three categories in my pie chart – my life is about work and home and I just don't have time to relax. Is that bad?

It depends entirely on how you feel about it as you look at the chart. Are you happy with things as they are? How do you feel about your life, knowing that one part of the chart doesn't appear in it? How balanced a picture is this to you? Just observe and consider.

Doing the pie chart makes me realise I am under a lot of pressure at home and it does affect me, but I think it's coming from other people and not from me. Do I still give it a big proportion?

Later on we will consider whether stress and pressure are created outside you or whether they arise as a result of how you react to situations. How big a proportion you give to the section on the chart is up to you; perhaps if you consider how much it affects you then you will be able to decide.

I find it really hard to just relax, I need to be doing something like going to the gym. Can that still count as relaxation?

Going to the gym is a very helpful thing to do for your health and well-being. However, if you lead a very busy life which makes you feel physically or mentally tired, then perhaps it would be useful to look at some other more relaxing techniques to use as well, to allow your body to recover and to improve your levels of well-being.

the physical side of stress

We are now going to take a closer look at how stress affects the human body on a physical level. You will have the chance to test your own reactions and see how big a factor physical stress is in your life. Learning more about your body's reactions is a great way to start managing stress because it teaches you how to observe certain signs and symptoms. Instead of living your life not realising what is going on, you can start to see yourself in a clearer light. This is the first major step towards helping yourself in the most appropriate way.

Stress and life events

When we feel as though life is going well, we can be busy, balancing lots of tasks and meeting lots of needs, seemingly without effort. This is the way we would like to feel most of the time. However, important life events do happen and they are major sources of reactions that we interpret as 'stressful'. Here is a list of life events that are generally considered to be very significant causes of stress. The most severe are shown at the top and the list decreases slightly in intensity as you work downwards, but all of these events can have a very strong impact, especially if several of them occur together.

- Death of life partner
- Divorce
- Marital separation
- Death in family
- Major illness
- Accident
- Wedding
- Major change in job
- Loss of job
- Moving house
- Retirement
- Change in work responsibilities
- Pregnancy/arrival of child in family
- Change in financial state
- Taking on a mortgage
- Relationship breakdown

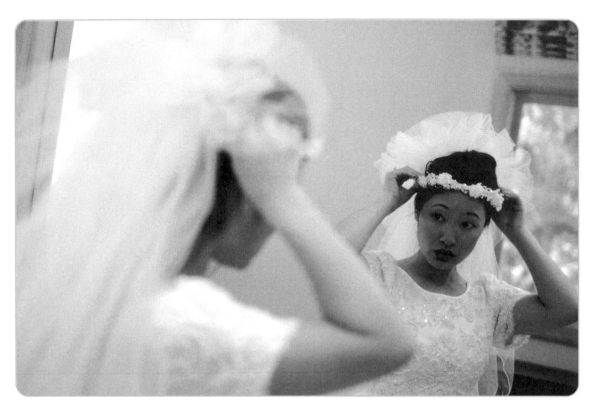

Weddings are often a source of a great deal of emotional tension

When you consider that we are all members of families, that many of us have life partners or long-term relationships, that we all have to live somewhere and that work is a key factor in all our lives, then this list starts to take on real significance. There is nothing unusual here; it is a list of very common life factors. We are all likely to experience at least some of them at one time or other.

Physical reactions

Events like the death of a person or sudden redundancy can cause a severe reaction, especially if they are unexpected. The shock of the news can cause the body's 'fight or flight' response to kick in immediately. Remember Chapter 1? This is the reaction which we saw in the first case study, when the prehistoric man ran for his life. It happens when the body is reacting to a highly charged life event. Physical changes happen very quickly; the breathing rate increases, the heart pumps faster, blood pressure rises and our arms and legs tense up as if to run, the muscles in them being primed with increased blood supply. Sugars and fats are released into the bloodstream to give us more energy instantly and, at the same time, other vital functions like digestion close down. The body is mobilised into flight mode; the adrenal glands which sit on top of the kidneys release hormones called adrenalin and cortisol, which prime the body into a heightened state. However, if all this readiness and energy is not used up in the physical act of running or worked off in some other physical way, then the whole body is kept in overdrive. Normally after a stressful event the body reverses the reactions by slowing the heart rate and breathing, lowering blood pressure, restoring blood supply to the digestive organs and relaxing the muscles. If the state of extreme over-stimulation stays in place, especially over time, then the body can start to show signs of damage; for example, high blood pressure, heart problems or depletion of the immune system, which defends you against infection.

In the 1950s Hans Selye, a pioneer of stress-related research, created what came to be called the 'adaptation curve'. This showed how a person reacts to a stressful stimulus from their environment, creating a peak showing what he called 'arousal'. This is what is going on when the 'fight or flight' response kicks in. Then there is a dip in the curve as the system reverts to a calmer state. Remember the exercise in Chapter 1? The prehistoric man showed a typical stimulation reaction to one stressful event. The modern man showed a different kind of curve, where the level of stimulation showed several peaks, meaning he was staying at that primed or 'pumped-up' level. As we have already seen, this could be the cause of further problems. Many people in modern times experience these repeated stress peaks and this can only deplete their body's resources.

One of the first signs of a physical reaction to stress is an increase in the heartbeat or blood pulse. If the body is at rest, the pulse rate is approximately 60 beats per minute. At times of moderate activity or stimulation it quickly rises to roughly 80–90 beats per minute. In an extreme situation, or, when the heart is working hard, the pulse rate could increase to over 100 beats per minute.

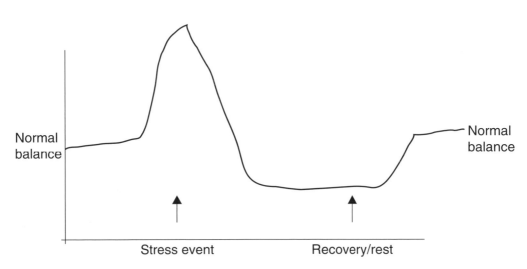

A single stimulation curve

stress management in essence

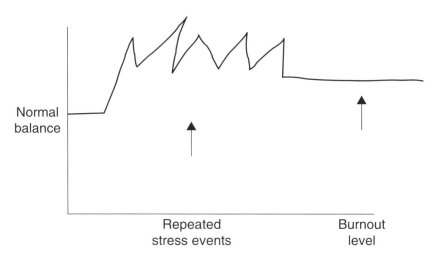

Repeated stimulation peaks

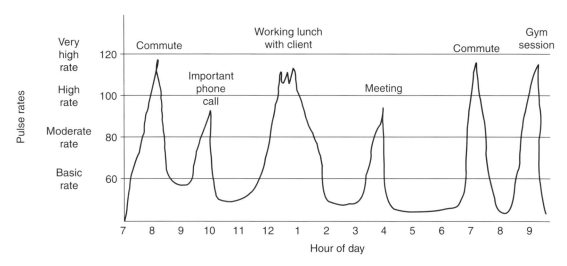

Heart rate peaks in a day

Above is another diagram to show some pulse-related stress peaks in a typical day at the office. Notice, for instance, that there is a major peak – where the heart is beating at over 100 beats per minute – very early on during the drive to work, and another one on the way home. Whilst getting your heart rate up to this level through physical exercise three times per week for 20 minutes is seen as beneficial to general health, getting over-stimulated and probably angry on the journey to and from work *every single day* is not helpful in the long run, and those emotions can put far too much stress on your heart. Commuting can be one of the most common regular physical stressors, creating feelings of anger and frustration, which translate themselves into a fast pulse reaction. Notice on this diagram the several other occasions during the day when the heart rate goes up. Look at the reaction to an important phone call or a meeting with a vital business contact. If you consider this pattern, which is by no means unusual, you can see how easy it is to experience physical heart-related stress. If this pattern continues uninterrupted for a long time you can see it could have more serious implications.

Take a few moments to think about a typical working day of your own and make a few notes about times when you notice you feel under pressure or perhaps experience an increase in your heart rate. How often do you think this happens? If the answer is regularly then you should talk to your doctor for helpful advice and also see if you can start to incorporate some simple relaxation exercises into your day, such as those we shall see in Chapter 4.

> Note – be aware that a sudden combination of symptoms like headache, dizziness or confusion and slurred speech are potential signs of a stroke; radiating chest pain or pain down the left arm are signs of a heart attack – both of these need immediate medical help.

Signs of physical stress

Let's take a look at some other examples of signs of physical stress in the body. This list is here to give you ideas of things to observe. Most of us regularly experience these types of symptoms in a minor way and we recover from them if we are allowed time to rest properly. However, if you feel any of these symptoms are happening to you regularly or severely then again it is worth getting advice from your doctor. Many physical effects of stress are relatively easy to deal with and some of the complementary therapies such as massage or aromatherapy can really help you to manage them better by 're-educating' your body to relax so it can restore itself.

Muscular tension linked to stress is very common indeed. People can hold stress-related tension anywhere in the body but one of the most common sites is the area around the neck and shoulders. If you are in a group, have a quick check among you to see how everybody's neck and shoulders feel, or squeeze your own shoulder gently with one hand to see for yourself. It is very likely that

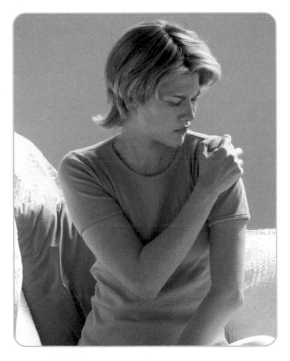

Muscular tension is a sign that the body is under physical stress

there will be a lot of stiffness – the area will feel hard and pressure will feel sore. Physical tension here can be due to bad posture, particularly when sitting at a desk or computer, but if there is extra stress due to external events the body may 'hunch itself' as a sort of defence. Regular body massage is an excellent way to loosen up tight muscles and improve blood supply to an area, making it more supple again.

Indigestion, diarrhoea and constipation are signs of imbalance in the digestive system; which, you will recall, is switched off during the 'fight or flight' stress response. If you overload your stomach with food while you are still in a primed state, then the digestion cannot cope, the stomach will produce too much acid and foods will not be broken down properly. This can lead to the stools being too loose (diarrhoea) or too hard (constipation), or can give you griping stomach cramps, which are signs of indigestion. This is why it is so important to eat in a relaxed atmosphere. It is not a good idea to eat if you are angry, upset or stressed. Persistent problems with digestion can show a significant underlying stress pattern that needs some attention; dealing with the cause allows normal digestive rhythm to resume. Often digestive stress effects are the result of emotions that have not been dealt with. Massage to the abdomen is a simple and soothing treatment that helps relieve tension in the area.

Physical exhaustion, where the limbs feel heavy and tired, can be the result of hard work such as gardening or DIY. Stress-related physical exhaustion is slightly different. It brings with it feelings of helplessness or futility – a sort of 'What's the use anyway?' type of question. It's as if you have been pushed beyond your limit and you just don't have any more to give. This kind of exhaustion occurs when you have been subjected to several of those severe life-stressing events in one go, such as getting a new job, being placed in overall charge immediately, feeling out of your depth and under pressure to perform. This kind of exhaustion needs attention; relaxation exercises and massage are once again useful techniques to help improve your physical energy levels.

Poor sleep patterns often happen because the body is so hyped up it simply cannot relax into readiness for sleep. This reaction often occurs because a person is caught in a loop of mental activity like going over and over the day's events, unable to 'switch off'. If someone takes work home all the time and never really ends their day, this can also impact on sleep. It's important to take a good look at your evening routine and check that you are giving yourself time to settle at the end of a day. Try to avoid watching late-night TV, or eating meals after 8pm to give your digestion a proper rest. A warm bath and some soothing music can be a much calmer way to help yourself wind down and get better-quality sleep.

Grinding the teeth or a generally tense jaw are both strong physical signs of stress. It is as if the mouth is clamped shut against something, possibly an emotional reaction which it may be helpful to bring to light. Constant tension here can have other knock-on effects like wearing down the teeth, or sending pain up into the forehead to cause headaches. Facial massage is a wonderful way to release tension in the jaw; you can either apply it yourself or, better still, have some treatment done for you. The combination of treatment and an honest look at what the underlying feeling may be can be most beneficial.

Headaches and migraines also deserve special mention; although they can arise for many reasons, such as poor eyesight, eye strain, food allergies or hormonal shifts, they are definitely made worse by emotional triggers or mental pressure. The physical effects of stress show up here as levels of pain, and in the case of true migraine this can be so violent that a person cannot bear to see light and may also be physically sick. If you suffer from either of these conditions regularly it is a good idea to talk to your doctor for advice. Complementary therapies like acupuncture (performed with needles applied to special points on the skin) or acupressure (pressure applied to the same points but with the fingers and hands) are very helpful to relieve pain.

RSI (repetitive strain injury) is a name given to an injury that has happened to the body where a particular area is suffering more than normal wear and tear. An example might be extreme pain and swelling at the base of the thumb because of typing. This example of a physical effect is linked to one of the other meanings of the word stress – remember, when so much force is applied to an object that it shows signs of breaking. Many repetitive strain injuries arise through work, especially if your job has a physical element to it. It's important to identify any problems as quickly as possible and get appropriate help to prevent serious long-term damage to the body.

So, summing up, we have just taken a look at a few of the most common signs of physical stress in the body:

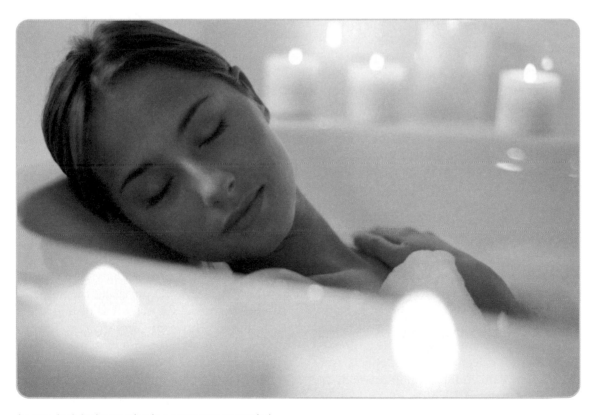

A warm bath in the evening is a great way to unwind

- muscular aches
- indigestion/diarrhoea/constipation
- physical exhaustion
- poor sleep
- grinding the teeth/jaw tension
- headaches/migraine
- RSI.

Write these down as a list and then next to them add two columns. The first column is for you to tick if you suffer from any of these symptoms. The second one is for you to write down how often – daily, weekly, three times a month, all the time. Again, a reminder – any constant or very regular problems may need some professional assessment and help.

This checklist of physical symptoms is a useful note for observation. In Chapter 4 you will find a wide selection of ideas to try to help you manage these types of symptoms more effectively. It can be very useful to come back to this list after a month or so of careful awareness of your stress levels to see if there is any direct improvement.

Next, let's look at a case study where the management of physical symptoms really helped improve quality of life.

casestudy

Sally is a teacher in a high school with a very busy schedule. She is popular with her pupils and with staff. One of her colleagues has been off sick for some time and Sally has had to take over some extra classes and duties to help cover. Although this was fine to begin with, now, after a month, Sally is beginning to feel very pressured. She is getting intense pain in her neck and shoulders and it's so bad that she has to take pain killers sometimes. She feels her neck is locked solid and she can hardly turn her head. She decides to have some massage treatment and, although that helps relieve the pain and tension, it does not go away completely. One day her massage therapist talks to her a little bit about why she may be stressed, and at that point Sally really offloads. It's as if all her resentment about taking on the extra work has been 'sitting in her neck'. Her massage therapist suggests she may like to talk to a counsellor about it, and Sally does. The more she understands why she is stressed and talks about it, the better her neck feels. She finds a way to express how she is feeling at school to her colleagues and her situation does improve – because she asked for help.

This example shows how feelings can really contribute to physical stress, creating tension in certain parts of the body. In Sally's case, getting some physical treatment helped part of the problem and then she addressed the underlying feeling, so the effects were even better. Pain and tension in the body are so often generated because of an inability to relax and let go. Sally got some much-needed help and her situation improved.

You are already seeing that it isn't really possible to separate physical, mental and emotional stress – they all interlink and affect each other. However, we shall go on in Chapter 3 to think about the mental and emotional aspects more deeply to help build up a more detailed picture of stress and its many facets.

FAQs

I am getting married soon – I thought that was supposed to be a happy occasion?

Well, I truly hope it will be for you; I think the reason why it is included in the list of stressful situations is that often weddings can turn out to be complex social occasions, with certain challenges when it comes to organising and paying for them.

How can getting pregnant be considered a major source of stress?

Well, again it depends on the circumstances; if a baby is anticipated and its imminent arrival is welcome that is one thing, but there may be other situations where the birth may cause shifts in relationships and other major challenges, maybe emotional or financial or both. These can be very testing for all parties.

Everyone experiences some tension at work, it goes with the territory – you are never going to have a stress-free job, are you?

Of course not, and the aim of pointing out job-related stress is not to suggest it can be eradicated, but more to highlight that its effects need strategies to help you deal more effectively with the pressure.

When I'm stuck in the traffic I do breathing exercises – I'm right in thinking this helps me?

Oh yes, definitely. Taking time to breathe slowly and regularly is one of the simplest and easiest ways to diffuse frustration and stress.

I'm a professional pianist and I'm getting lower back pain. It worries me and I think that's making me even more tense. What should I do?

Get yourself assessed, possibly by your doctor or by a qualified sports therapist or osteopath. You will need some professional help to correct your posture and ease any muscular spasm you are feeling. Also, try some of the relaxation techniques in Chapter 4 to help diffuse your anxiety.

I've heard that Indian head massage can really help headaches. Is that true?

Yes, provided you receive it from a qualified practitioner. The treatment works on your scalp neck, shoulders and arms and eases out tension all over your head.

stress, the mind and the emotions

We are now going to consider how stress affects the way you think and feel, changing how you react and behave. In many ways, these highly important aspects of mental and emotional stress often underlie the physical manifestation of problems – they tend to be there in the background and, unless they come to light, then physical problems can persist. As we have said previously, exploring these inner aspects of stress does not mean you have to lay bare your soul, particularly if you are working in a classroom as a member of a group. The exercises in this chapter are designed to show up patterns for you to observe and consider. How far you decide to work to change them is entirely up to you. In Chapters 5 and 6 you will find many different ideas to help you with simple techniques to manage mental and emotional pressure. You can easily adapt these to everyday life.

It's important to say here that we all feel mental and emotional stress; It's a fact of being alive in this place and time. There is no magic wand that will make these feelings go away and, besides, would we really want to live like robots without emotions? Of course not. Our feelings and thoughts allow us to interpret and react to the world around us in every moment of existence. They are vital and valuable tools that can help build our perception of how the world is. The emphasis we are looking for is *balance.* If feelings and thoughts get out of harmony then the picture we see of the world becomes distorted, and that in turn creates more disharmony, more distortion, and so on. Managing mental and emotional stress is very much a question of identifying key thoughts and feelings, noticing the kinds of effect they have and choosing to work with them differently. Sometimes you can do this on your own. However, if the pattern you identify is too complex or severe, then it is good to seek professional guidance. Therapy has a vital role to play in helping people identify their issues and find ways to feel empowered to cope with them. You will find details of different kinds of professional approaches to counselling and other branches of psychotherapy in 'Where to go from here'. This book is meant to help you explore the idea of mental and emotional

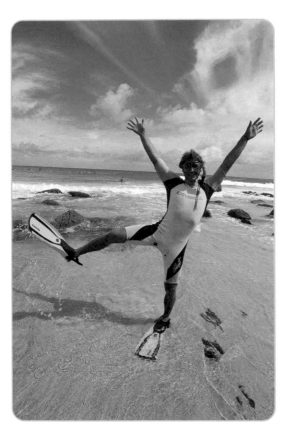

Our feelings and emotions express how we react to our world

stress in a simple way: it is not intended as a course of therapy.

Mental stress is something that often arises out of a complex combination of events that together present an overwhelming picture. Take learning to drive as an example. How baffling it all seems at the beginning – learning what all those sticks and buttons do, getting the hang of steering, feeling how the car moves – all that, plus dealing with situations on the road and reading signs . . . it can easily knock you off balance. I recall a day when I was out practising with my brother and I 'lost it' – the road situation was too much to cope with and I just stopped in my tracks, my mind went into stress overload and I panicked. Thankfully, I got past that and am now fine with driving, but I remember that combination of events very clearly.

Mental stress and overload

Here are some common signs of mental stress and overload for you to consider.

A racing mind is one of the key signs of mental stress. It means your thoughts are flying through your head at an incredible pace and nothing gets to completion. Thought patterns are more like a flood and they do not help you make useful choices. This mental state is often associated with insomnia; the mind cannot switch into sleep mode because it is replaying events over and over. If you are under extreme pressure then it is easy to lose your sense of 'centre', a balanced place inside

where you feel calm. Breathing exercises and meditation techniques are very helpful to learn and apply on a regular basis to improve the situation, as you will see in Chapter 5.

Finding it difficult to concentrate is connected with this racing mind – of course, if thoughts are flooding through then it becomes very difficult to focus on one thing at a time. Concentration is like a laser beam, it pulls a lot of mental power together to apply it to one situation or challenge. It can be quite an effort to do this anyway, particularly on a sustained basis, and even more difficult if you already

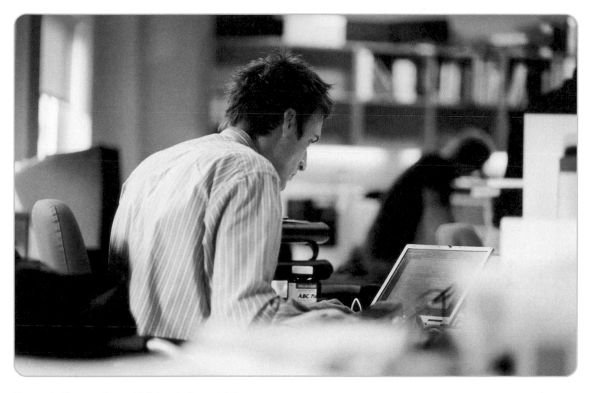

Concentration requires a high level of mental focus

feel muddled. This is why regular breaks are a good idea where you get some fresh air and breathe deeply to clear your head.

Forgetfulness is something we all feel momentarily, none of us is perfect! However, if you are constantly finding yourself forgetting things and this causes disruption in your life, then there is probably a mental level where you are not connected to the present moment, so you are not noticing important things. For instance, if you keep finding bruises on your leg and you forget when they happened, that is an example where you have actually hurt yourself but you have been so disconnected you didn't notice. It's very important to learn techniques to ground you in the present moment. Then you will notice things and remember them.

Being unable to take in new information is often a problem people think is due to their level of intelligence. However, although it could be the case that the complexity or depth of the information is too much for a person to understand, often an inability to absorb new things is a sign that what has come your way has arrived too quickly, too intensively or at too large a volume for you to take in. It takes a level of self-discipline, but you can learn to break things down into bite-sized chunks to help you absorb key information.

Rash behaviour means taking unnecessary risks with a kind of 'Who cares?' attitude, placing yourself and possibly others at risk. This kind of attitude may be a kind of call for help or a cry for attention. Being rash is acting blindly with no thought for the consequences. This kind of pattern is a deeper one and may well benefit from professional guidance.

25

Getting over-fussy happens when the mind is so overloaded that a person latches onto particular things and goes over and over them again and again, showing signs of extreme impatience with others. In a work situation this could be a sign of great mental insecurity over performance, so a person rigidly sticks to what they know. It is as if this person is stuck in a loop of their own making, and they need support to break the pattern and feel confident to take on something new.

This list is not exhaustive but it gives you an idea of some of the most common signs of mental stress. Experiencing any of these patterns does not mean you are 'unstable', but they are important clues to what may be affecting you in the moment. It is helpful to notice how intense they are and how often they affect you. As we saw previously, there is a kind of 'day-to-day' level where these kinds of behaviour will arise where you recognize them and cope with them easily. Where they become more intense and constant, then that may be a sign that you need to work with a professional to learn to deal with them more constructively.

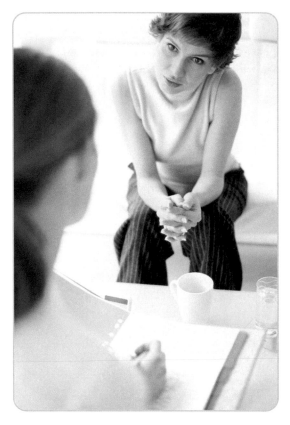

Talking things through with a professional is helpful when problems are complex

Exercise

In your notebook, write down any of these signs of mental stress that ring a bell with you. Using a scale of 1–10, where 1 means no effect and 10 is extreme, see if you can assign a number to show how intensely you think this pattern affects you. Then write down how often you think this pattern occurs, whether it does so in a particular area of your life – e.g. work, home, family, relationships or environment – and why this might be.

For example:

Situation	Value	Happens	Link	Why?
Forgetfulness	7	Most of the time	Family link	So much going on I can't keep track

Identifying an area like this can show up something you can choose to look at and work towards improving. As a start, ask yourself how you would like to be supported to improve this situation.

If you are working in a classroom group, perhaps you could compare notes in pairs or small groups to work your ideas through in more detail, being careful to support each other with respect.

Emotional stress

Our emotions or feelings are another aspect of the overall picture of stress. Emotions are literally 'e-motions' or 'energy in motion'; they are powerful and can strongly influence our lives, sometimes bringing change incredibly quickly. Falling in love is an example. It brings headiness and a view through rose-coloured spectacles, life instantly looks brighter, and

nothing matters but the person you love. Hopefully this is a positive example of emotion, but of course as we all know there are negative emotions too. These tend to cause emotional stress which can affect us very deeply to the point where life becomes almost frozen and we experience emotional pain or even numbness. Emotional stress patterns are

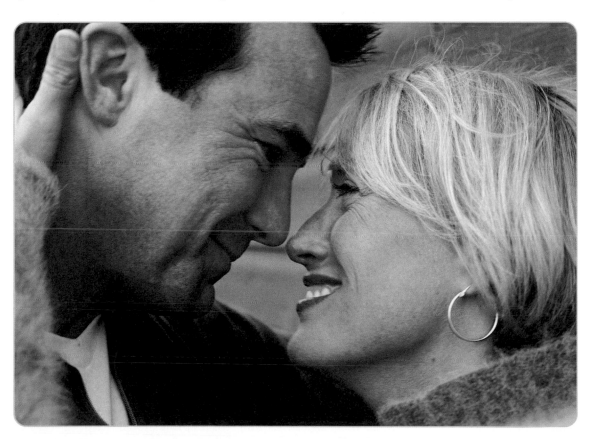

Emotions like falling in love are very powerful

some of the deepest and most complex manifestations of stress, often at the very core of what is going on, and unravelling them can benefit from professional help. Again, it depends very much on the intensity and duration of the feelings.

Other important things about emotional stress patterns are that they tend to arise out of interactions with other people and often have their source in childhood. If you were constantly told you were useless, and your talents were never acknowledged as a child, this may have significant effects on how you feel about yourself as an adult. Events that knock you backwards may generate thoughts like 'Well of course I can't do it', and bring about feelings of depression or futility. However, these thought patterns can be changed, and by building your own sense of self-worth you can choose to see yourself differently. Later on in the book we will look at some ways to start doing this.

For now, let's have a look at some of the most significant signs of emotional stress.

Depression is an enormous topic and the subject of many volumes of discussion and research. It includes feelings of sadness, hopelessness and often a loss of interest in life. Of course, we all experience these feelings from time to time, but if they occur regularly they may be a sign of a deeper problem. Fits of crying for no apparent reason, mood swings, loss of appetite and sleep problems can be signs of underlying depression. Clinical depression – diagnosed by a medical professional – is the most common psychiatric condition and it is estimated that between 10–15 per cent of the population suffer from it during their lifetimes. Statistically it is more common in women than in men, but this could be because women generally find it easier to talk about their issues or to seek help, while men are conditioned to cope by 'putting on a brave face'. Also, many women suffer from depression triggered by lifestyle and hormonal shifts after childbirth – post-natal depression. Depression can be medically treated using antidepressant drugs. However, personal exploration of issues is important too, to help build confidence in a person to develop coping strategies in their own life. This is where professional help is important (see the section 'Where to go from here' at the end of the book).

Anxiety is a form of fear that can immobilize a person and totally influence their life. We all feel anxious at times, but usually these feelings pass. A person in a severely anxious state will entirely shift the way they function when faced with the idea that something they dread will happen. For example, some people can become too afraid to go outside – a state called 'agoraphobia'– because they fear a particular set of circumstances. Symptoms of severe anxiety go back to the 'fight or flight' response – a pounding or irregular heart rate, tightness in the chest, an inability to breathe deeply and a dry mouth are common signs. Being reassured by other people will not change a severely anxious pattern; a person needs support to grow in self-confidence so they are able to make decisions based on a more positive outlook.

Phobias – like agoraphobia mentioned above – are extremely powerful but limiting behaviour patterns based on a very specific belief that something is a threat. There are many kinds; for example, claustrophobia is an emotional stress reaction to enclosed spaces like lifts, arachnophobia is a fear of spiders. Depending on their intensity and duration, these types of emotional reactions may require some professional help to change

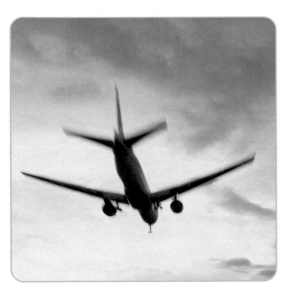

Fear of flying is common and there are courses to help you overcome it

them. It depends on how intensively they affect a person's life.

Panic/panic attacks – these are signs of extreme emotional pressure, often accompanied by heart palpitations or rapid breathing (hyperventilation). Mostly they are triggered by what seem threatening or fearful situations, like fear of flying. Relaxation exercises and deep breathing techniques can be very helpful ways to cope with them. However, it is important to identify the cause to really stop them happening.

Feelings of abandonment or isolation are signs of emotional stress which may have roots in early childhood. They can lead to very withdrawn behaviour, affecting a person's relationships with other people. If someone holds a deep-rooted belief that they will always be abandoned then they will never trust anyone to stay with them and they will always be alone. This kind of stress pattern is one that really does need some professional support.

Reading a list like this can be quite a depressing thing to do in itself, but it is only there as a general guide. If we look back at the last two chapters, we can see that it's quite easy to get in touch with how stress affects us physically and do things to help ourselves. If our minds are experiencing feelings of overload there may be a need to look at the circumstances of our lives and see if some improvements are possible, or perhaps we need to learn some new tools to help us cope. Although we can sometimes deal with negative feelings ourselves, there may be times when we feel overwhelmed and getting support from a professional may be the way to go.

Sometimes it is easier to consider mental and emotional stress patterns in context. Here are two real examples of reactions to the same situation, which occurred some years ago when I was working in human resources. I had two men to deal with who were approaching retirement. They were approximately the same age and were due to leave work at exactly the same time.

stress, the mind and the emotions

casestudy

The first man, let's call him Pete, was very sociable and well-liked in and out of work. Although he had loved his job he had always maintained a balance of sporting and social activities outside it. When it came to his approaching retirement, he was looking forward to it, had made lots of plans and was feeling very positive about it.

The second man, we'll call him Mark, was totally absorbed in his work to the exclusion of anything else. He always worked long hours and his colleagues teased him about not wanting to go home. He had a wife and family and, as far as we knew, all was fine there; it was just that Mark was completely work-focused. When it came to thinking about or planning his retirement he didn't even want to contemplate it, and at the leaving party he was very withdrawn.

The following Monday, after both men had left, Mark came back into work. He couldn't cope with the idea that he had retired. It was very strange and awkward for managers to go and talk to him. They had to convince him that his working life had finished. Sadly, Mark went into deep depression and three months later we heard that he'd had had a stroke and was very ill. It was very unfortunate.

Consider these questions:

1 If you look at these two scenarios, what do they tell you about how Pete and Mark dealt with the life-changing event of retirement?

2 There is no doubt that it is a stressful time, when you have to start seeing yourself differently beyond your work. Pete already had that sorted out for himself, but Mark found it much harder. Why do you think that was?

3 Even without knowing the full circumstances of Mark's life, some aspects of his situation are still very evident. What kind of conclusions do you think we need to learn from these two men's reactions?

It is important when you are dealing with mental and emotional stress to understand the signs and also the intensity of what is going on. Everyday ups and downs are one thing, but deeper, more persistent patterns are important to identify and these may require you to work with someone professional to guide you. It is a great pity that Mark was not able to avail himself of such help.

FAQs

How do I know when it's best to get professional help?

In any situation, when you get to a stage where you know you can't deal with it on your own, that is a point where professional help would be a good thing. Actually, identifying this stage and seeking that help is a major step towards better self-awareness and understanding.

I've got my parents-in-law coming to stay for the first time and I go into a state of complete panic every time I think about it. I just freeze. What can I do?

Firstly, perhaps talking it through with your husband would be a good idea. Why is this so daunting for you? It is important to share your feelings with him. Then maybe enlist one or two close friends to help you plan the time and make a checklist of things you need to do to make sure all is prepared.

I'm usually fine when I'm asked to concentrate, except if it's on something I don't want to do. Then I let anything distract me. What can I do about this?

Well, it depends what the thing is that you don't want to do and why this is a problem for you. Maybe that is the level you need to look at and talk to someone about. If your fear is linked to not being able to perform a task, then you need to identify why that is. There may be lots of ways to get the support you need to get the skills you need.

I'm approaching my menopause and I notice I get very strong mood swings, especially with my hormone cycles. Why is this?

This is more likely to be due to hormonal changes, and it is a good idea to talk to your doctor to get appropriate help. Relaxation exercises and regular practice of techniques like yoga can be very helpful to help your body cope with the changes.

Can phobias be 'cured'?

Yes, if a person is prepared to face whatever their worst fear is. Not facing the fear is usually the cause of the problem. This is easy to say but more complex to achieve, which is why things like severe agoraphobia – fear of going outside – may need professional guidance. Some airlines run special courses to help people overcome the fear of flying. There are many ways to deal with phobias.

I think all this talk of 'professional help' is a waste of time. Sometimes you just have to take what life throws at you and get on with it.

Well, fair enough if you think you can do it. However, some people find themselves in circumstances they feel they can't deal with on their own. Putting on a brave face or ignoring what is going on can actually cause more problems in the long run.

how to deal with stress patterns

This section of the book looks at simple and practical ways to cope with physical, mental and emotional stress. You will find a whole range of tools to try which are designed to be easily incorporated into your daily life. Start using a few today and you will really see a difference in your energy levels, and also feel improvements in your own sense of well-being.

relaxing the body

As we have already seen in Chapter 2, physical stress patterns are relatively easy to identify for yourself. They often relate to sensations of tiredness and lack of physical energy. A typical sign of physical stress in the body is waking up feeling tense or just as tired as when you went to bed, even though you may have been sleeping for several hours. If any of these feelings apply to you, or you feel tension in a particular part of your body, then you can try some of these simple techniques to see if you can improve the situation for yourself. In this chapter there is a wide selection of ideas to try; you can use them in a classroom situation to experiment and compare notes with your classmates, to find out what feels good to you. They can also just as easily be tried if you are working through the book by yourself, though it can be fun to get a friend to work with you as well. Exchanging ideas and sharing experiences is a great way to learn.

Two things are apparent when you start using these techniques. One is that *they take some time*, which means the pace of your day immediately slows down. However, we are not talking hours here: each one may take 10–15 minutes to do. You may be surprised at how long a time that can actually feel. Using just one or two techniques a day takes very little out of the hours you spend awake, but knowing you can 'take time out' in a constructive way to help yourself is a huge psychological boost.

The second important thing is that *many of these techniques use touch*, that is the simple application of hands to the body over clothing. Touch itself is a vital sense in the management of physical stress. Think back to childhood; if you fell and hurt yourself, how important were the reassuring hands of a caring adult in helping you feel better? If you are physically or emotionally stressed, a simple caring hand on the shoulder can make all the difference. It is a pity that as a society we have become somewhat wary of touch because it can be misused, and if it is in any way forced on someone then that is a level of abuse. However, if it is offered sensitively and in a respectful way, then touch remains one of the simplest and most effective diffusers of physical stress. It actually lowers blood pressure, reduces the heart rate and encourages the whole body to relax.

What is relaxation? It is not laziness, being idle or doing nothing. Nor is it necessarily sleeping. As we have seen it is perfectly possible to sleep and wake up tense. If we go back to that

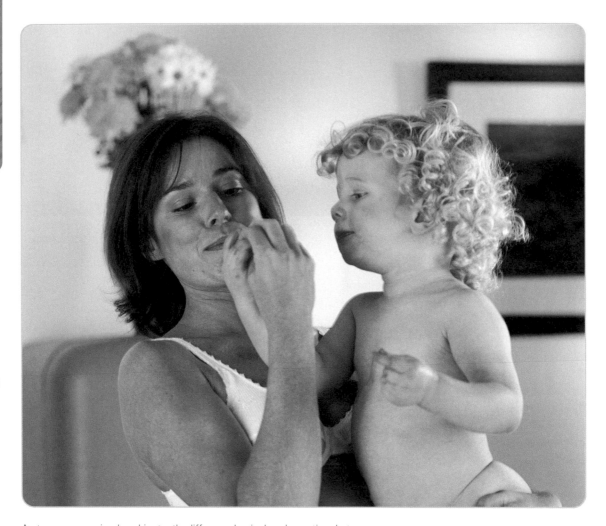

A strong reassuring hand instantly diffuses physical and emotional stress

original idea of 'fight or flight', the point at which the stimulation curve dips back down again is when the body goes into a relaxation response. This is due to a change happening within the nervous system where the brain emits a different set of chemicals that counteract the stress response by allowing blood back to the organs as well as to the digestive system. This reaction also allows the body to rebalance itself and encourages renewal at cellular level. The breathing rate slows down,

blood pressure lowers and the body rests. If we stay in the heightened stress pattern too long, the body never gets the chance to relax properly and restore its energy levels.

Here are a selection of different exercises to choose from to help you experience a sense of deeper relaxation and calm. They fall into several groups: first, exercises done lying down; then standing or sitting; then using a technique called 'palming'; and finally a set for the feet. Choose the ones that appeal to you and try them. With the exception of one of the foot techniques, all the other exercises are designed for you to apply to yourself. Each one takes about 10–15 minutes. You will see that many of the exercises involve breathing techniques. Combined with simple stretches and movements, controlled breathing is one of the most effective ways to diffuse and ease physical stress.

Exercises in a lying position

For these exercises it is useful to place a blanket on the floor and fold it in half to make a comfortable surface to lie on, or you can use a yoga or exercise mat if you have one. Wear comfortable loose clothing and socks to make sure you stay warm.

Stretch and Release Sequence

Lie down on your back with your arms and hands resting slightly away from your body. Breathe gently and regularly a few times and feel your body settle onto the floor. Now

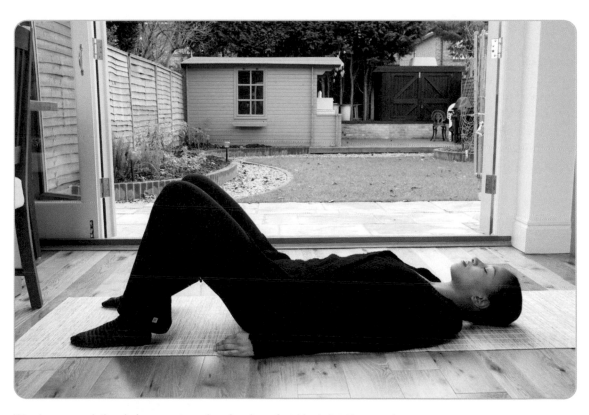

Wearing warm clothes helps you stay relaxed and comfortable during the exercises

stretch both your feet down and away from you for a few seconds, then let them relax. Then stretch the whole of your left leg for a few seconds, and relax. Repeat with your right leg. Moving up, stretch both your hands away from the body and then relax them. Then stretch your left arm for a few seconds, and relax. Repeat with your right arm. Now move up to your shoulders, and hunch both of them up towards your ears, hold for a few seconds, then relax. Turn your head from side to side a few times, then come back to the centre. Now be still, relax and notice how your body feels. A lot of physical stress is carried in your arms and legs. This exercise shows you the difference between being tense and relaxed.

Inner Circular Breathing*

This exercise requires you to lie on your back again, in a comfortable position, arms away from the body and legs slightly apart. If you want to cover yourself with a shawl that's fine; it's important to stay warm. Take a few deep breaths and relax. Now, breathe in and when you exhale, imagine a line of light which travels from the crown of your head all the way down the front of your body to your feet. As you inhale again, imagine that the line of light continues under the soles of your feet, up the back of your legs, up your spine and onto the top of your head again. Then exhale again, slowly, and send the light back down the front of your body, and as you inhale, imagine it travelling up the back of your body. Do this a few times until you can really sense a circular pattern of light flowing down the front and up the back as you breathe. After a few moments, just breathe normally and notice how your body feels.

Hand on Head, Hand on Abdomen

Start by lying in the same relaxed position as with the previous two exercises. This time, place your right hand on top of your head. (You might need a cushion under your arm to support you.) Then place your left hand over your abdomen, on top of your navel area. There is no need to apply any pressure, just rest your hands in these positions. Breathe gently and regularly. Stay like that for a few moments and notice what happens to your body. You may feel warmth under your hands, a sensation like tingling, or even a feeling of energy passing up and down your body between your hands. This is a very simple energy-balancing hold typical of traditional Eastern healing methods. Try it for 5–10 minutes at a time. You can also use this exercise in bed at night to settle yourself before sleep.

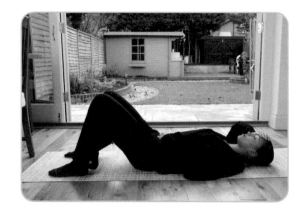

This simple position is deeply relaxing and can help prepare you for sleep

*This exercise needs to be done slowly.

Exercises in a standing/sitting position

These exercises require you to stand, or to sit comfortably on a dining chair. The standing exercise is really effective if you do it outside in the fresh air. For the sitting exercises it is good to have a window open because fresh air is so beneficial in all these exercises involving breathing techniques. As before, warm, loose clothing is advised.

breathe in, lift your arms slowly out to the sides and bring the palms of your hands together over the top of your head. As you breathe out, slowly bring the hands back down to the sides of the body. Repeat this exercise 6 times, slowly, really stretching the arms out, up and down each time. Then come back to the starting position and notice how your body feels.

Standing – Breathing Exercise

Stand with your legs shoulder-width apart, your arms loosely at your sides. Breathe normally a few times to centre yourself. Now as you

Sitting – 9 Calming Breaths

This is a sequence of breaths that you count. 9 is a special number; because we work in units of 10, 9 is the last number before the beginning

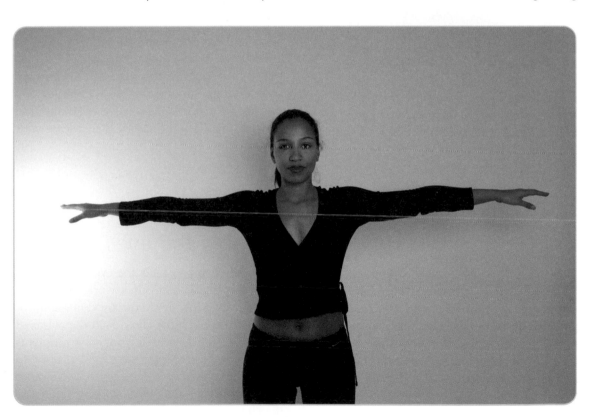

This exercise strengthens your arms and deepens your breathing

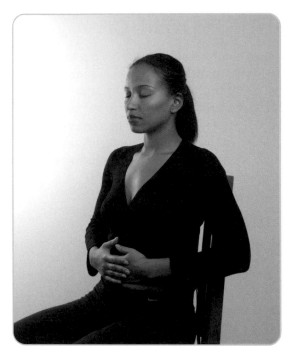

Wait for the heat to gather under your hands – this feels very soothing

another. This sequence of 9 breaths is very useful if you suddenly feel physically tense – it helps you end the cycle of tension and open yourself to a new phase. Sit comfortably and close your eyes. Breathing in and out counts as one breath. Start counting down from 9 to 1. This is easier for concentration. Watch what happens to your body and breathing as you count. See how you feel afterwards.

Sitting – dissolving tension with the breath

This exercise is very useful if you feel there is tension concentrated in one part of your body – for example your abdomen. Many people feel tense here when they are anxious. Sit quietly and place your hands over the area you feel is affected, here the abdomen. As you breathe, imagine there is a warm golden light building under your hands. Once you can visualize or feel it, then imagine this light spreads into the area of tension and, as you breathe, any discomfort just dissolves. Keep breathing into the area for a few moments, then release your hands. Notice how you feel now.

of a new cycle. In numerology, the study of the significance of numbers that goes back thousands of years, the number 9 is a symbol of the end of one phase and the beginning of

Palming exercises

Palming means rubbing the palms of your hands together really briskly then applying them to your body. What this does is literally 'charge up' your hands, a bit like charging up iron filings with a magnet back in school. Your body has an electromagnetic field around it and rubbing the hands together simply energises them. Applying them feels very soothing. You can do palming either sitting or lying down.

Palming the eyes

This really helps to relax the eyes, especially if you do a lot of computer work or have to concentrate a lot, or if you are doing a lot of close work like embroidery. Rub the palms of your hands together briskly for a few moments then just rest them over your eyes. It's best to close your eyes while you do this as it's more relaxing. Your hands will feel very tingly. As the charge decreases, repeat the process. Your eyes will feel very rested afterwards.

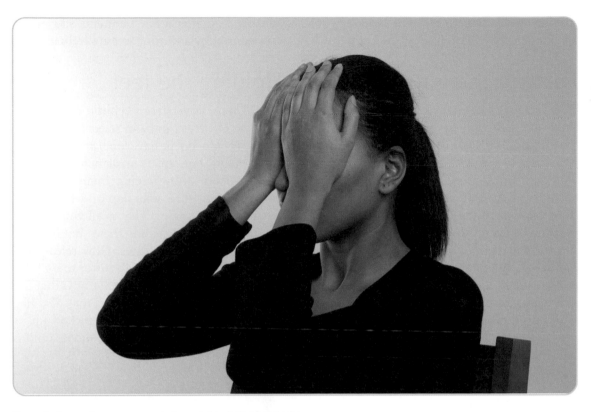

Eye palming really eases eye strain and also helps headaches

Palming the lower back

This is a 'quick fix' for lower back tension, particularly after sitting for long periods. As before, rub the palms of your hands together, then apply them to your lower back. Feel how warm they are, and notice that warmth spreading into the area. Again, the charge will diminish, so repeat the process a few times. It is surprising how quickly you will feel relief.

Foot exercises

The feet are a very neglected area of the body and it is a shame that so many people seem to dislike their feet so much. They are a vital connection to the earth, to ground and centre us in the moment. Many spiritual traditions

Palming the lower abdomen

Here the same technique is applied to the abdomen, and the tingling palms will help ease tension as well as spread warmth into the area. This application is also good for any discomfort such as indigestion or cramping pains.

like Buddhism place great emphasis on the feet making contact with the ground as a way of diffusing physical tension and bringing a sense of inner calm. Bare feet are best for these techniques. If this a challenge for you I would still encourage you to try. The soles of your feet are sensitive in more ways than you think.

Feet touching the earth

This exercise is one where you need to stand barefoot, preferably outside and actually on the ground. If it's too cold outside you can try it indoors. As you stand there, really spread your feet wide, move your toes so you feel anchored. Let your arms be relaxed at your sides. Now as you breathe in, imagine you are drawing in energy and light from the sky, the sun and the stars. As you breathe out, imagine this energy runs through your body, out of the soles of your feet and down into the earth. Keep breathing in energy from above and sending it through the body, out of the feet and into the earth. All the time your feet are your

anchor. Stop after a few moments and notice how your body and your feet are feeling.

Holding the feet

This exercise is very simple but it does need a partner. The feet can be in socks for this one. Here, all you do is have one person sitting comfortably, perhaps in an armchair, and the other person sitting facing them. Lift your partner's feet onto your lap and hold both feet under the ankles. That is all you have to do. Just keep your hands there, holding the feet, for about 10 minutes. Now release the feet and tell your partner to lower them back to the ground. Ask your partner how that felt and listen to the feedback. You may also like to share any impressions you picked up as you were holding the feet. This simple hold is

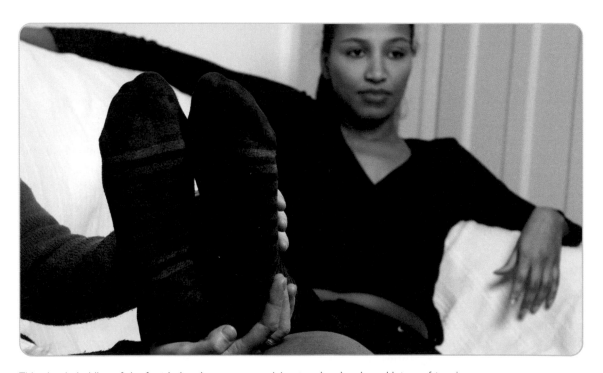

This simple holding of the feet helps the person receiving to relax deeply and let go of tension

incredibly physically relaxing; it calms and soothes the whole body. It's very useful to apply to children who have difficulty sleeping.

Summing up, we have covered some simple exercises designed to calm and ease physical stress symptoms in daily life. As we have said previously, any regular signs of physical discomfort that don't seem to improve should be referred to your doctor. None of these exercises will do you any harm, but if you notice any persistent patterns of physical stress it is in your best interests to get some professional advice.

Here is an example of how these exercises can be incorporated into daily life.

casestudy

Julie is a busy woman who is a marketing executive for a software company. She leaps out of bed at 6.30am each day, rushes into the shower, dresses and grabs a quick coffee before leaving the house at around 7.30. She then has a stressful drive to work, where she is on the go from the moment she gets to her desk. Meetings, presentations, dealing with clients – she sails through her day. She enjoys her work but the pace is very fast. She has to eat as she goes along, and she often does not get lunch unless she eats with a client. If she's lucky, she gets home at around 7pm after another long drive.

She's noticing some signs of physical stress. Her eyes get very tired, particularly towards the end of the day. She wears contact lenses so the problem it isn't with her eyesight itself; it's the concentration. Her shoulders are very tense from driving and from sitting at a desk. She's also having trouble getting off to sleep at night, even though she feels exhausted.

Have a look at Julie's day and see if any of the techniques shown in this chapter might help her. What do you think?

We suggest Julie could include eye palming at regular intervals during her day to help her eyes. This only takes a few minutes and allows a brief interval of calm. She could use the tension-dissolving breathing exercise, too, in a break, applying hands to her shoulders. She could also include the energy hold of one hand on her head and the other on her abdomen to help settle her into sleep at night.

In the end, we live the lives we live; techniques and simple exercises like these help us to deal with the challenges of the day.

FAQs

I always feel guilty about relaxing, I feel like I'm being lazy. Is this unusual?
No, a lot of people feel this way. It comes from the old 'Victorian work ethic', which dictates that not doing anything is unproductive. Actually, it's the opposite. People who can balance activity and rest are more productive.

How often should you do the exercises?
As often as you feel you need them. However, if you are just starting I suggest you choose two initially that appeal to you, and try them for a week: one in the morning and one in the evening. At the end of the week, sit down and write a few notes about any changes you feel in your body.

I do a lot of exercising in the gym – isn't that supposed to help physical stress?
Moderate levels of physical exercise can relieve stress, but if you are already tired and physically stretched pushing yourself even more may not be doing you a lot of good. The suggestions given here are very gentle and are introducing you to the idea of relaxation as a way to recharge your batteries.

When I do the Inner Circular Breathing I feel really warm afterwards as well as relaxed – is that OK?
Yes. This breathing exercise comes from the East and is used in many traditions. It is a way of regenerating the energy of the body at core level, so feeling warm shows that it is working.

I find I really enjoy the exercise with one hand on the head and one on the abdomen, but I seem to fall asleep while I do it – is that OK?
Yes, it's fine. It's a sign that your body has deeply relaxed. You should find that your sleep feels a lot more refreshing as a result.

Someone made me really angry at work the other day, I felt sick, but I remembered the 9 breaths – it helped so fast. I felt really different afterwards – is that usual?
I'm glad it worked for you! Yes, if you use the best tool at the time you will see quick results – as you did here. Making a choice like that and helping yourself in the moment is a great way to manage physical stress.

refreshing the mind

Mental stress affects us all at one time or another. It is a state where the mind feels totally overloaded and all our usual coping mechanisms seem to disappear, leaving us in a state of confusion and even helplessness. Mental stress is often connected to lifestyle issues around work or family and is accompanied by a feeling of 'build-up' over time. However, there are ways to cope with these stress patterns to keep a better internal balance.

In this chapter we will have a look at some of the situations that affect mental stress in more detail, and then we will explore some simple techniques to help manage them. These ideas can be practised in your classroom group to get you used to the way they work, or you can try them on your own. The key to success is using them regularly. Trying something once and then dismissing it immediately will not help you; trying a technique out for a week or more and then looking at the results is more realistic. The good news about the mental stress management tools used here is that none of them require a great deal of time. If managing time is one of your pressures, you will be pleased that you can easily incorporate these techniques into your daily life without disrupting your routine too much. However, once you start to feel some benefit then you may decide to take a look at how you are running things and to make some changes.

If we recall what was said in Chapter 3, key signs of mental stress are things like a racing mind, difficulty concentrating, loss of focus, or inability to take in new information. These may be accompanied by physical symptoms, too, like a racing heart, sweating, damp palms or stomach cramps. The body is showing signs of being in a state of high alert, and if this is not alleviated, then over time the effects may be more serious; for example, increasing the risk of damage to the heart.

Many people feel mental stress in connection with their work. Recent scientific research has discovered that stress is one of the main reasons why people take time off work. In many cases employees feel totally overwhelmed by demands that they cannot meet or helpless because they have no say in how work is to be managed. They may be pressurised to produce quick results and judged negatively if they do not, or feel that their managers give them no support. One in five workers report feeling stressed at work, which equates to approximately 5 million people in the UK. Given that claims for compensation for

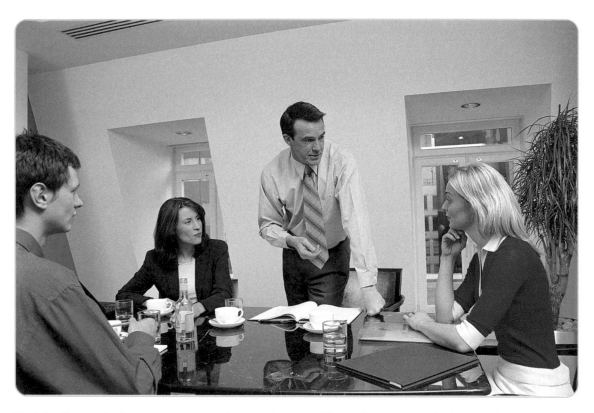

Tight deadlines and extreme pressure to perform are factors which contribute to stress in the workplace

work-related stress are on the increase, it would seem to be in the interest of companies to address ways to improve the working environment of their employees by decreasing levels of occupational stress. However, even though stress is a factor against which employees in the UK are covered under the Health and Safety at Work Act of 1974, any preventative measures companies might take are still optional. The levels of consultation, training and improvement in relationships required to make large-scale changes may be seen as very costly to organisations in terms of time and money. However, some companies do work in a consultative way, creating good communication channels and opportunities for collective problem solving. These measures help employees to feel included in the dynamic processes of the workplace, and this eases workplace stress.

One of the most important aspects of occupational stress seems to be dealing with the issue of powerlessness. If you work in a place where you are overwhelmed and you feel unable to do anything about it, this will be a key factor in mental overload. However, even if your work situation is difficult and you do not feel you have any power to influence it, if you can turn that situation around and realise that you can still make *some* choices, then you can start to reclaim your personal power in the situation. Putting it simply, 'if you can't change the situation, change yourself'. This is actually taking a more spiritual perspective along the lines of traditions like Buddhism, where the way the world seems on the outside is less important than how you are on the inside. If you can get in touch with a place of peace and 'centre' within yourself, this is one of the most potent tools for dealing with any external situation, no matter how difficult it may seem. What happens is that from the place of 'centre' the situation may actually start to look different, and the way you react to it will change. This can unleash a new set of events that are more likely to take you forward.

Meditation

This is a tool that is really worth learning as a first step towards managing mental stress. It is a way to calm the mind and find inner stillness. Regular practice also encourages a better breathing rate and even changes one's brainwave patterns to a more relaxing cycle. Some people take to meditation very easily and others have to practise it like a skill, but over time it gives you real benefits in terms of mental relaxation. Ten minutes in the morning and again in the evening is a very helpful practice to develop. This will help to calm and centre you at the beginning of your day and help you 'switch off' at the end of it.

There are different techniques you can try and it is worth experimenting to see which one works best for you. The best position for meditation if you are new to it is to sit upright on a hard backed chair with your feet parallel on the ground and your hands resting loosely in your lap. You may like to put a shawl around your shoulders to keep you warm. In the East where meditation is a regular practice, sitting cross-legged on the floor is more common.

Here are three examples of techniques; each one is designed for a 10-minute session.

Breath focus

This is one of the first and simplest meditation techniques. Here you don't need to count breaths or make them particularly

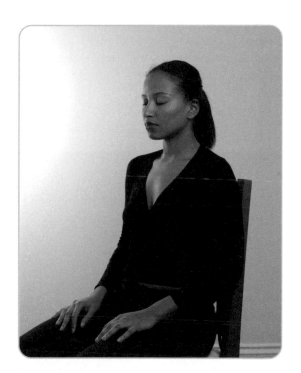

Sitting on a hand-backed chair gives you an upright posture which is perfect for meditation practice

deep, just maintain a regular breathing pattern in and out. Just focus on that pattern, listen to your breath going in and out. Relax in the chair, sit and breathe. If thoughts come in, imagine them in soap bubbles you can just blow away; if your focus shifts, guide yourself gently back to the breath. After 10 minutes, stretch, and wriggle your toes. See how your mind feels now.

47

Candle focus

A technique that lets you concentrate on a single object, in this case a candle flame. Sit on your chair with a table in front of you, with a candle in a holder in the middle of it. The flame itself is a source of stillness. Focus your attention on the flame and hold it in your vision as long as you can. If your attention drifts, bring yourself gently back to the flame. Notice all the colours it contains. After 10 minutes or so, stretch yourself a little and notice how your thought patterns feel.

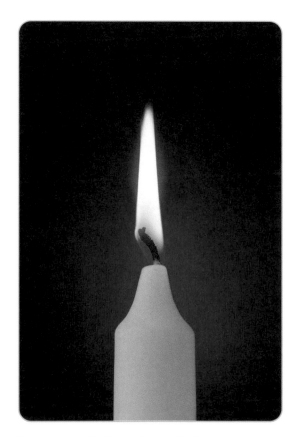

The beauty and stillness of a candle flame helps to calm the mind and focus the thoughts

Mantra focus

A technique used in India and other Eastern countries, where certain words are said to carry a special vibration. One of the simplest and most powerful of these is 'OM', which is a word that means many things, including peace. Sitting comfortably on your chair, choose a note that is comfortable for you to intone, and make the sound 'OM'. Repeat it slowly, taking a deep breath each time. Listen to the sound of your voice in the stillness making the sound of 'OM'. After several repetitions, notice how your mind and body feel now.

Visualisation

Another technique to use to try to improve your sense of mental well-being. It involves sitting in the same position as for meditation, but instead of working with different levels of focus, you use your powers of imagination to visualise certain types of picture. This technique really suits people with an active imagination who have no difficulty 'seeing' at an inner level. The images suggested here are simple and use colours with a soothing effect on the mind. If you want, you can record these visualisations on tape so you can listen to them as you focus. Pause between each sentence to allow yourself time to create the image.

A Rainbow of Colours

Relax in your chair, take a few deep breaths, feel yourself sitting comfortably. Close your eyes. Now visualise a warm red colour in front of you. Really experience the rich abundance of this colour, luminous with ruby red lights. Next, a rich bright orange shade, warm and cheering. Then see this change to a lustrous golden yellow, glowing with light. After this the colour changes to a rich vibrant green,

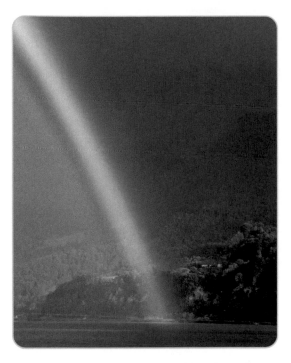

Colours of the rainbow make up a vivid palette of shades which soothe the eyes

you can use this picture if you wish, or you can create a new one in your imagination.

You are standing on the shore of a beautiful peaceful lake. The water is still, and reflects a perfect sky above so the colour of it is a deep, restful blue. It is so calm that you can see all the trees around the edge reflected perfectly on the surface. If you look up, you see beyond the line of trees to a mountain in the distance, capped with snow. The summit gleams in the sunlight. The mountain gives you a sense of strength and helps you feel grounded, you feel your feet on the earth and you know you are safe. As you continue to look at the mountain, you see a bird flying towards you, and as it reaches the lake its reflection glistens on the still surface of the water. Its feathers gleam with gold from the sunlight. You watch the bird and it gives you a sense of freedom and peace.

Stay with the picture for a few moments, then take a few deep breaths, stretch, and let the image dissolve. Notice how your mind feels now.

Rose in the Heart

This image is particularly soothing to use if you are suffering from a combination of mental and emotional stress. The rose is a symbol of love and beauty, and its fragrance is one of the most evocative of all aromas.

Visualise a beautiful rose in bud just about to open. You can choose the colour you want; maybe deep velvety red, lush pink, warm apricot, golden yellow or pure white. You will instinctively know which shade is right for you. Once you have chosen, imagine the flower before your eyes. As you watch, it begins to open, each petal unfurling, soft and gently fragrant. When it is fully open, really focus on the beauty of the whole flower. Feel the softness of the petals, inhale the perfume,

emerald-tinted and full of life. Now it moves to the colour of a summer sky, a deep shimmering azure blue. Then the colour deepens even more to the indigo blue of a night sky, soft and calming. Finally, it changes to deep violet, a shimmering amethyst hue.

This ladder of rainbow colours is vibrant, and each colour holds a meaning for you. Spend a few moments going through the colours again or, if you wish, focus on one colour in particular that appeals to you at this time. Let yourself be nourished by these colours.

To come out of the visualisation, take a few deep breaths, stretch, and wriggle your toes. Notice how your mind and thoughts feel now.

Mountain Lake

This visualisation uses geographical images. If there is a particular mountain lake you know,

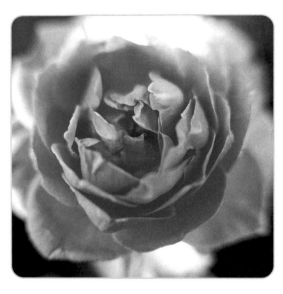

The rose is a beautiful flower which symbolises peace and love

see the beautiful shade of its colour. Then imagine that you can put this flower into your heart. Let it sit there, spreading its light and fragrance, and feel your mind and emotions grow calm, soothed by the presence of the rose.

Stay with the image for a few moments, then take a few deep breaths and stretch, letting the image dissolve. Let yourself continue to be relaxed and notice how you feel now.

You can return to these visualisations any time you need them. After each one you may like to make a few notes about anything you saw or any feelings that seemed important.

Yoga

Yoga is another amazing tool to help mental stress; it involves special stretches to the body. The word is from the ancient language of India called Sanskrit, and it means 'union'. There are different individual positions called 'postures' in yoga, with names like the Plough, the Fish or the Forward Bend. Yoga is a practice which brings mind and body into harmony; concentrating on the posture is a way of bringing discipline to the mind. There are different branches or types of yoga, and the best way to incorporate it into your life is to join a regular class. However, if you would like to try some simple postures yourself, here are four examples. To perform yoga exercises it is best to wear loose clothing like a tracksuit. Work on a soft surface or on a yoga mat if you have one.

> Note – with all these stretches do not force any movements. Only go as far as you feel comfortable. If you have any back problems then it is best not to try yoga on your own; you need a qualified teacher to advise you.

The Cat

To prepare for this posture, kneel down on the floor on all fours. Breathe regularly and easily.

First, as you breathe in, slowly arch your back upwards as far as feels comfortable and look down at your hands. Then as you breathe out, relax the back down slowly and push your hips up as far as feels comfortable, also

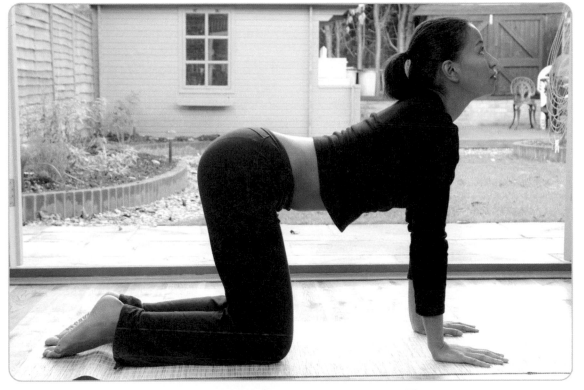

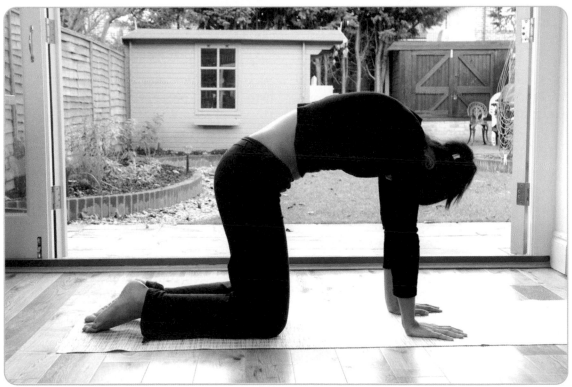

51

The Cat posture gives a gentle stretch to the spine and the abdomen and is good to ease stiffness after sitting for too long

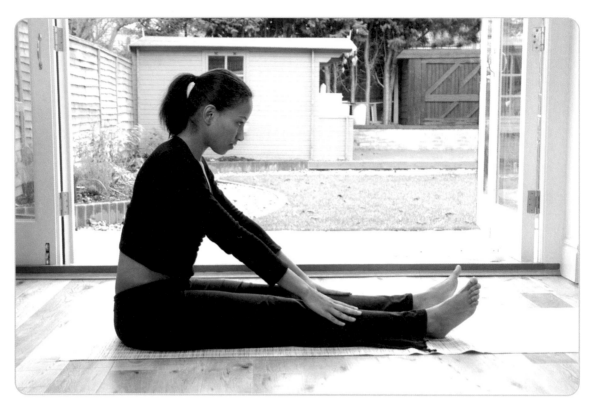

When you lean forward don't overstrain, go as far as you feel comfortable

stretching your neck and looking upwards. Repeat twice more, slowly, noticing your breath as you do so.

The Sitting Forward Bend

To prepare for this posture, sit on the floor with your legs stretched out in front of you. Sit with a straight spine and your arms loosely by your sides. Breathe regularly.

Breathe in and lift your arms up to either side of your head. Now exhale and bend forward slowly from your hips, leaning over so you reach down your legs with your arms as far as you can. Don't force this stretch; go as far as feels comfortable. Breathe regularly and stay in the stretch for a few moments. Then breathe in, and as you exhale slowly, come

back up to the sitting position again. Repeat twice more.

The Cobra

To prepare for this posture, lie down on your stomach on the floor with your arms bent so the palms of your hands are flat on the ground at shoulder level. Breathe regularly.

Inhale, then as you exhale slowly, push down on your hands and stretch your arms, thus raising your torso off the floor. Look upwards. Keep your legs in contact with the ground. Go as far as you can, hold for a few seconds then release the arms slowly and bring the top half of your body back to the starting position. Relax for a few moments, then repeat the sequence twice more.

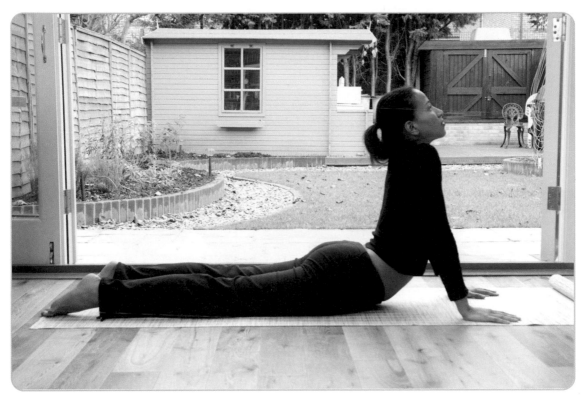

Stay in the posture for a few moments; your arms may tire and start to shake a little – if so come down again slowly

The Child Posture

To prepare for this posture, kneel on all fours and breathe regularly.

This time, as you exhale, come down to the ground, bringing your knees up to your chest area and lowering your shoulders, resting your forehead on the floor. Let your arms curve loosely around the sides of the body. Continue to breathe regularly into the posture, which is very relaxing. Stay there for a few moments.

This little sequence of four postures takes about 15 minutes to do and is a great way to unwind at the end of a stressful day.

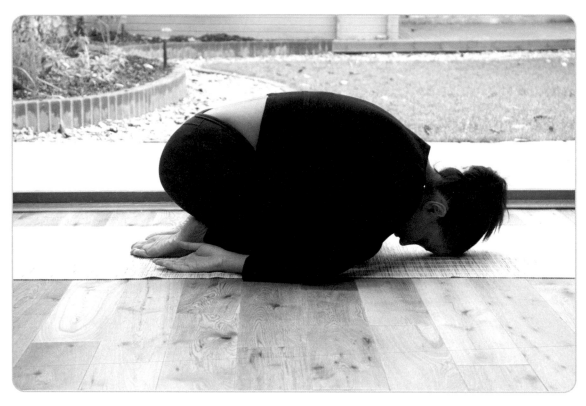

Relaxing in this posture helps to ease out the spine as well as soothing the digestive organs. It also feels very calming.

case study

Ben is a good example of someone who has taken meditation to heart. He used to be very mentally driven, often running around trying to do several things at once. He's a fit man of 43 but he had a scare a few years ago when mental stress pushed up his blood pressure. Then he took a course in meditation and it really changed his attitude. Now, not only does he practise mornings and evenings for about 30 minutes at a time, but he has also started to take 10 minutes during his lunch break to centre himself, and he uses breathing techniques before he has to go into potentially stressful business situations. He has also started to learn Tai Chi, a Chinese art which improves energy levels and mental awareness. As he says, 'I've realised managing stress is really about finding the tools which work for you and using them regularly. I love my meditation practice and I think it's improved me as a person.'

Following on from Ben's account, have a think for a few minutes and make a few notes of how you could create for yourself a simple mental stress management plan. Choose one activity for the morning – a meditation, a visualisation or the yoga posture sequence – and another for the evening. Make a commitment to practise this plan for a week, and note how you get on.

As Ben discovered, managing mental stress can actually open up new levels of awareness and empowerment. Instead of being swallowed up by pressure, taking some responsibility changes how you react to the external situation. Your level of internal balance can directly affect your external experience – for the better.

FAQs

I get mentally stressed at work and sometimes I feel really angry because I'm not being listened to. What can I do?

The anger is part of the frustration at being powerless. If you try to express yourself while you are angry, you may do more damage to the situation. However, if you practise some breathing or some meditation techniques to centre yourself, you may well find that you can communicate how you feel in a more constructive way.

Isn't meditation like mind control?

It depends what you mean by 'mind control' – if you think it means somebody else taking over your mind, then that is not at all what it does. Meditation helps you get better at directing and focusing your *own* mind, which is a very different thing, and helps you to think more clearly.

When I try any of the meditations I just can't focus for more than a few seconds. What can I do?

Try the grounding the feet exercise from Chapter 4 to start with, to get yourself very centred in your body. Take some nice deep breaths before you begin. Then just be patient; if you can concentrate for 10 seconds to begin with, that's fine. The more you practise, the more your focus will increase.

I'm amazed that seeing the colours in that rainbow visualisation makes me feel so energised. Why is that?

The rainbow colours make up the 'colour spectrum', which is the range of colours visible to the human eye. Science shows that each colour carries a vibration: tones like red, orange and yellow are warmer; and green, blues and purples are cooler. Working with the visualisation is giving you an experience of the energy levels of the colours.

Do I have to practise all four yoga postures in one go?

Those four postures have been chosen to make a short 15-minute routine to fit in with the day. They also stretch and bend the spine in a carefully complementary way. For best results, they should all be done together.

How can I find out more about yoga classes?

Consult your local adult education centre or look in your local paper, the Yellow Pages or the Internet, where you will find classes advertised. Make sure that the instructor carries a yoga teaching qualification.

understanding
your emotions

As we have seen so far, there is a range of different techniques that you can apply to help yourself through stress as it manifests itself on a physical or mental level. These levels are quite simple to identify and you can improve those patterns quite quickly by incorporating a few simple measures to change your daily life. However, if you recall what was said in Chapter 3, sometimes the physical or mental manifestations of stress are caused by deeper emotional feelings. While we all have emotions and feelings that enhance our lives by allowing us to express ourselves, they also have the potential to do so positively or negatively. If negative emotional patterns are left unresolved over a long period of time, they can lead to more constant states like depression or anxiety. Then there may be physical or mental stress signs that link to the underlying emotional pattern. This is a more complex situation that may require professional support.

It is important to emphasise again at this point that this book is not intended as a course of therapy. Whether you are using it in a classroom situation or on your own, it works only at a very simple and basic level, introducing some ideas for you to work with either in your group or by yourself. If you decide you want to explore these ideas in more depth or you have deeper issues, then have a look at the 'Where to go from here' section at the end of the book, where you will find details of actual therapeutic approaches that may help you.

How can we deal with our emotions ourselves? Is that possible? Aren't feelings just moods that happen to us and we can't do anything about them? These are valid questions to ask at this stage. As we have said before, to feel is to be human. Perhaps the thing to bear in mind is that we can't stop feelings occurring and nor would we want to, but we can start to observe them and understand them a little differently. If we can learn to apply more observation to ourselves, we become more self-aware, and then we can choose – if we wish – to consider different ways to react to situations. Emotions are directly linked to behaviour; they influence every aspect of life. In their positive role they

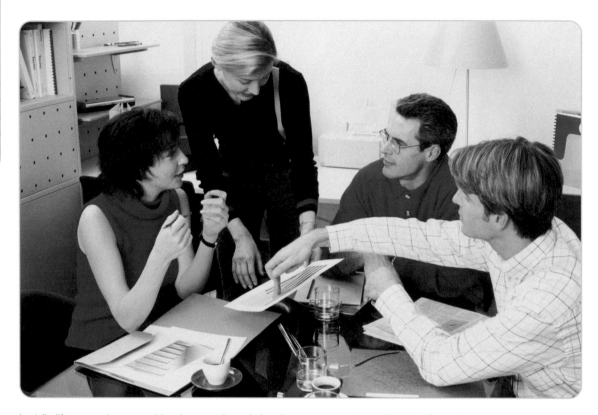

In daily life, as we interact with other people and situations, we experience all kinds of emotions

allow us to express how we feel and enhance our experience; if they get out of control or start 'running the show', then we may begin to find life events reflect our inner level of imbalance.

It may be a challenge to you to consider that what is going on in your life is always down to you. Nobody else is responsible. You make the choices you make, instant by instant, you choose how you react to situations every single day. You may think that 'they' or 'someone else' or 'he' or 'she' are responsible for what is going on for you, but they are only reacting to a situation as they perceive it, just as you are. How you choose to respond is always your choice whether it feels conscious or whether it's a gut reaction. You have still decided. If you are a person who tends to react with powerful emotional outbursts and find that people respond in the same way, that is a pattern to observe. After working through this chapter you might want to consider if you would like to change how that behaviour pattern works for you . . . because you can. Then, you can begin to live your life in a state of understanding, not at the mercy of overwhelming feelings. This does not mean you become a robot. Instead, it means that you are learning to act from a place inside you that is wiser and more aware.

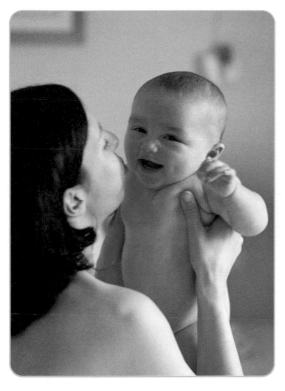

Our lives are filled with the expression of feelings fuelled by our emotions – how we behave is directly linked to how we feel

Cognitive behavioural therapy

In this chapter we are going to explore some approaches to observing and understanding emotional patterns in a very basic way. The techniques we are going to use are simple examples of techniques along the lines of cognitive behavioural therapy, or CBT. This is one of the most effective approaches to deeper psychological work currently in use. CBT is a very rigorous and scientifically monitored way of dealing with emotional patterns, and to experience it fully you really need to follow a course of therapy with a CBT qualified therapist. However, there are some basic principles that can be understood and applied

more simply, and this is the level we shall explore here.

To understand what CBT is, it helps to summarise its history. In the early twentieth century, Sigmund Freud and other pioneers of psychological therapy created the concepts that underpinned psychoanalysis up until the 1950s. They worked on the premise that the roots of all dysfunction lay in childhood and offered analysis to help work with these patterns. However, this approach tended to be very expensive and only available to a select few. From the 1950s and 60s another group of techniques were developed called

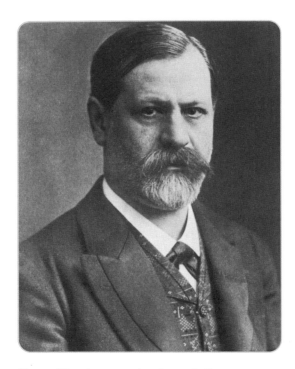

Sigmund Freud was a major pioneer in the development of psychology and psychoanalysis in the early part of the twentieth century

'behavioural therapies', which made deeper psychological analysis more widely available. These approaches, broadly speaking, worked with the symptoms of anxiety and incorporated the idea of 'learned behaviour' patterns that could be changed. Then, in the late 1960s and 70s, an American psychiatrist called Professor A.T. Beck spearheaded the development of a treatment for depression called 'cognitive therapy', which emphasised the role of people's thought patterns in the development of depression. These two approaches have merged to become 'cognitive behavioural therapy'. This takes into account the fact that particular thought patterns are associated with particular emotional problems. Unlocking these means helping the mind to reassess and re-evaluate how thinking affects behaviour. In a professional context, specific CBT techniques have been developed over the years and scientifically monitored to show effectiveness in situations like addictions and eating disorders, as well as a wide range of anxiety disorders. This is where professional guidance is absolutely essential.

Learning self-assessment

We will begin by adopting simple techniques along some CBT lines. This requires some work from you. You will be asked to think about and assess situations and feelings in some detail, and it is important to be honest with yourself. There is no judgement here; the process we are working through together is simply showing you how to become more self-observant. This is a skill you are developing that can serve you very well in your life, and like any skill it can take time to learn. If you can approach the exercise with an open mind and a willingness to find out more about yourself, then you will appreciate the benefits.

Collecting and recording your data

This approach to understanding an emotional pattern requires you to collect some data. To do this, in your notebook you need to create a record of an aspect of your emotional life and keep it going for a week. Try to write down notes under the headings shown below, each time you experience this emotion, as near to the event as you can. Remember, don't judge yourself – you are just observing.

Sit quietly and have a think about how your life is generally at the moment. Is there a persistent negative emotional feeling that is coming up for you regularly? It could be anger, frustration, fear, worry, doubt, anxiety or whatever becomes apparent as you take a few moments to focus on what is going on. You are invited to choose to observe one emotional pattern more closely over a week and learn when, how and why it is affecting you.

In your notebook, write down the following:

Emotional feeling: I am choosing to observe . . . . as it arises in my life for the period of one week from (date) . . . . to (date) . . . .

Each time the emotion comes up, as soon as you can write down some notes under the following headings:

Date and time: these are important to record, especially if the feeling happens more than once a day. Remember to write notes each time the feeling occurs.

Situation: here you state briefly what was going on at the time when you experienced the feeling; where you were, what happened and who was involved.

Effects of the feeling: how did the incident leave you in terms of your emotions? Give it a value on a scale of 1–10 for intensity, 1 being virtually nothing and 10 totally overwhelming.

Body sensation: did you notice any signs in your body at the time? Again, give any sensations a value on a scale of 1–10 for intensity, as above.

Here's an example of how an entry might look:

Emotion: fear

Date and time: 3 Dec, 10.30am

Situation: Dental appointment, hate it, really get scared it might hurt

Effects of feeling: value 6, anxiety is quite intense before the appointment

Body sensations: dry mouth, stomach cramps, value 7 pretty intense for me

---

stress management in essence

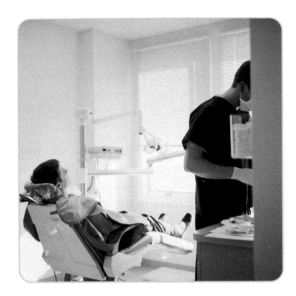

When you go into a situation you think will be fearful, what do you find? Is it really as daunting as you think?

As you can see. you don't have to write a lot, just simple notes, but you do need to make an entry in your record each time your chosen feeling comes up over the week-long period.

After a week, stop writing the entries and take some time to read them through carefully. You may start to see some patterns emerging already – similarities in situations that keep coming up.

Now let's take a closer look at the feeling you have been exploring.

Consider these questions:

1 Is there any evidence for my feeling?

For example, if you are observing fear levels in yourself, what was the actual evidence that there was anything to fear in the situations you logged? Did events actually happen to bear out your fears? Check each of your entries and add a note on this.

2 Is there any evidence against it?

Here, observing the same emotion, was there anything that contradicted the need for it? For example, if an event you feared did not happen, this is evidence shows your fear was not necessary.

3 Is this feeling helping me or not?

Look at the pattern of occasions where this emotion has occurred and consider – does it improve your life or not? Sometimes fear is a useful thing, it might stop you from stepping out in front of a car. Sometimes it may not be helpful if it holds you back from experiencing something important in your life.

Check the entries you made using these three questions:

- Did events bear out my fears?
- Was there any need to feel the emotion?
- Did the feeling help me or not?

You may be coming to some conclusions already. If so, then make a few more notes. Now let's take a look at how you could start to work differently with this emotional pattern. In your notebook, write down the following statements that you are going to fill in as an overview of your data entries.

My feeling is . . .

This feeling impacts on my life by . . .

I know this feeling is going on because . . .

Sometimes this feeling helps me by . . .

However, sometimes it's not helpful because . . .

If this feeling has an advantage it might be . . .

However, its disadvantages are . . .

A more realistic way to help myself to deal with this feeling might be. . . .

If we use the fear example, you might end up with something like this:

My feeling is fear.

This feeling impacts on my life by making me scared to try new experiences.

I know this feeling is going on because my mind races, my heart beats fast and I want to hide.

Sometimes this feeling helps me by protecting me from danger.

However, sometimes it's not helpful because things I think might be dangerous or scary turn out not to be so.

If this feeling has an advantage it might be that it does protect me sometimes.

However, its disadvantages are that it really holds me back from trying out new things and it limits my life experience.

A more realistic way to help myself deal with my fear might be to try one or two things that seem less daunting and see how I get on, so I build up my confidence.

Once you can see an overview of your emotional pattern, you are ready to try out your new awareness of it in a safe way. That is why the last statement in the list is significant. It is important in the next immediate period of time to try out your new awareness and notice how you are responding. Treat yourself gently and with respect – nobody is asking you to be superhuman. For example, if you

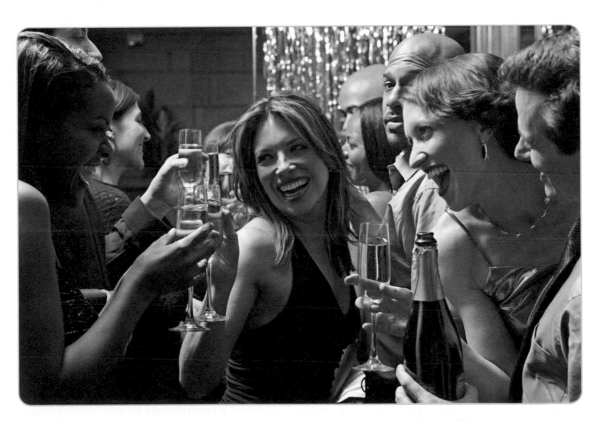

Dealing with your persistent negative feelings can open the way for new enjoyment in your life

are dealing with fear over going to a party and talking to strangers, talk to a sympathetic friend who will introduce you to a few people, go along, and see what happens!

Here are some other suggestions you could use to monitor your progress:`

ॐ Reread your entries from time to time, especially if the same situations come up again – have your observations and reactions changed now you are more aware of the pattern? If you give number values to the intensity of your reactions, have these changed too?

ॐ Watch out for any physical signs of stress associated with this pattern – how often do they come up now? As time goes on they will hopefully start to decrease, which is another positive result for you.

ॐ Congratulate yourself – even treat yourself to something rewarding – when you do something to meet your challenging emotion and deal with it successfully!

ॐ If you try a strategy and it doesn't work, be gentle and don't over-criticise

yourself. Sit quietly and consider why it might have happened. Was there evidence that you attempted too much this time? How do you know? How could you approach this situation differently to help yourself?

When you are dealing with persistent emotional patterns in your life you will not be able to change them overnight. You are not expected to suddenly transform everything as if with a magic wand. These techniques can help you to start observing your reactions more carefully – this alone can be a powerful way to illuminate your understanding of yourself. With time and some patience, you may begin to notice moments in your life when your awareness starts to pay off because that is when events around you show signs of changing for the better. The feeling of achievement when this happens is very supportive to you; suddenly you may realize that you have a lot more choice in your life than you ever thought before. This is when you begin to live your life from a point of self-responsibility rather than simple reaction.

FAQs

I have a tendency to blurt out whatever comes into my head in emotional situations and sometimes it gets me into trouble. Can the methods here help me?

Yes, if you are prepared to be patient and go along with the steps that are recommended. The fact that you can identify this pattern in yourself is interesting – you could apply the techniques to this and see what level of understanding you reach about it.

I can't see myself stopping every time I get my feeling and saying, 'Oops, sorry, have to go and make some notes' – it's just not practical!

Well, you don't have to do that – just keep your notebook to hand and see if you can make a note as soon as possible after the event. The idea is to note it so that over time a pattern emerges that you can see and understand for yourself. You may find you always behave in a certain way in certain situations, which you did not even realize, and this may be something you find you would like to change. The information you collect is important to help you complete the exercise and learn more about yourself.

I am a very calm person normally – I still think it's other people who get on my nerves and cause me problems.

If this is your perception, then I'm not here to argue with you. However, you could ask yourself, if you are so calm, why you get irritated by 'them'. Why docs 'their' coming into contact with you cause you to feel this way?

I can't identify just one feeling to work on in the exercise – I feel there are several coming up, all roughly equal. How do I choose which one to work with?

Allow your intuition to guide you. Let these feelings work through your mind and the one that needs the most attention will present itself. You will know which one it is and it is important that you choose it for yourself. Sometimes understanding one feeling like this can unlock the others, too, along the way.

It's all very well analysing everything like this, but what good is it going to do in the long run?

The analysis is only there to help you gain a better understanding of how, when and why you react to situations in a certain way. You don't have to analyse for the rest of your life – you are here to live it – but learning more about your own patterns of behaviour can really be of benefit to you and those around you. In the long run this can help you to respond to situations without becoming overwhelmed by your feelings, which means clearer decision-making as well as better levels of understanding.

I've always had a tendency to have a very short fuse. I get angry very easily. I'm a bit worried about noting this down – what does this say about me?

I'm not here to judge you, nor is anyone else. Whether you are working in a classroom group or whether you are on your own, how much you choose to share your conclusions is up to you. The exercise is not designed to point a finger at you and make you feel guilty; you are who you are. If you are noticing the level of anger you feel, that is a useful step; looking at the pattern it presents via the exercise may well support you to make some changes that ease that pressure for you.

lifestyle factors and stress

We have now explored ways in which stress affects the body, the mind and the emotions. Stress as a subject is now taking on a different meaning; we know it is a word that is simple to say, but as an idea it already covers many different levels. At this point we need to consider other elements that can be influenced by the impact of stress on our lives. These are called 'lifestyle factors', and they revolve around important areas of our daily existence. In this chapter we will take a closer look at some key factors, to learn more about them and what they can mean to us. This is valuable information because some of these factors may need to be changed to reduce our stress levels. Lifestyle factors relate to choices we make on a daily basis about what we eat, drink or take into the body. These factors can be affected by our stress levels because they relate to things we choose to put into our bodies to influence how we feel.

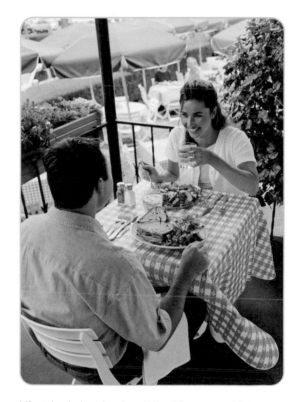

Lifestyle choices involve all the things we put into our bodies, and the balance of the effects these have together

Assessing lifestyle factors

Again, as we have said previously, this material is not designed to point a finger at you. The information can help you to assess your own lifestyle factors so you get a better picture of elements that may be causing you extra stress. It is useful to have a look at your own life and think about the factors we will discuss. If you can do this honestly and consider what the information means to you, then you can make a more informed choice about any changes you think may be beneficial to you. Nobody is here to judge you; only you can decide what is right for you. It is always your choice. These days, in magazine articles and in the media, there are certain concepts which are bandied about as popular 'dos and don'ts'. These messages are often oversimplified and easy to misinterpret. If you are considering any major changes to your lifestyle habits it is always wise to consult your doctor first for support and guidance.

The most important thing to assess with lifestyle factors is the intensity of the effect. Some factors are relatively harmless in moderation, but if you get to a point where you can't do without something then you are looking at a potentially addictive pattern that can affect your body over time. Addictive patterns of behaviour are more problematic to break because the body is conditioned to the 'reward' of the act itself, and therefore a habit is set up which becomes a potentially harmful loop. A craving that is always satisfied creates another craving, so when you look at personal lifestyle factors it always helps to ask yourself, 'Could I take this factor out of my life easily and still feel fine?'

Stress patterns contribute to the picture because they very often trigger the craving.

A really common example is a situation of mental overload, confusion or difficulty 'staying with it', so the impulse is to reach for coffee. Coffee contains caffeine, which is a stimulant. It gives you the illusion of more energy, but in fact it sets up a negative loop that depletes you even more so you need more coffee … and so on. Emotional stress issues like depression may lead to more serious cravings for alcohol, for example, to 'numb' feelings of negativity. However, this will not take the emotional issue away. It is estimated that at any time one in ten people will be suffering from depression of some kind. The temptation to try to make it go away by using some form of compensation such as alcohol is a trap that many people fall into. They may not even consider themselves to be depressed. They may not even recognise the signs. These days, behaviour like 'binge drinking' is on the increase, and perhaps in your group or on your own you may like to take a few moments to consider why this might be.

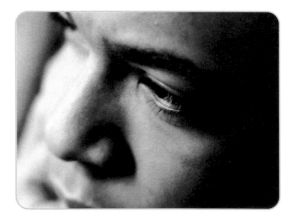

Feelings of depression can lead to certain cravings to help compensate for stress or to numb our reactions to it

Key lifestyle factors

Let's take a look at some key lifestyle factors. We are going to examine them in two groups:

1 Common dietary factors that have limited effects if used in moderation but which can easily become addictive at high levels. (Nutrition and stress is a huge subject and I do not propose to go into it in depth; if you want to study it further then I recommend another title in this series, *Nutrition in Essence* by Sarah Bearden.) However, we will look at some basic ideas here.

2 Factors with stronger potential to become addictions, and which need careful monitoring. Becoming more aware of them means you can choose to take measures to support yourself.

Common dietary factors

Sugar

We are born with a taste for sweet things; one set of taste buds on the tongue is designed to pick up this sensation. However, research has shown that the more excessively sweet tastes are given to infants and small children, the higher the craving for sweet things will be in later life. The body does need some sugar to convert into the energy we need to function and move our muscles. We can convert this successfully from grains rich in carbohydrates – like oats, for example – but this is a slow process. In the moment when we 'need energy' it is very easy to reach for something that contains refined sugar, such as fizzy cola-type drinks or sweets, chocolate or biscuits that give us an 'instant high'. However, blood sugar levels go up very fast in this instance,

and the body will not be able to use all of the intense input. The excess will tend to be stored up as fat. It is a good idea to monitor the amount of refined sugar you take into your body over a few days; notice not just what you eat or drink but when, and how often, and most important *how you feel* when you think you must have it. If you notice a pattern of reaching for sugar when you feel stressed and emotionally low, then perhaps this is an area you need to investigate more closely to discover what is really going on. The need for sugar may well be masking a deeper emotional need.

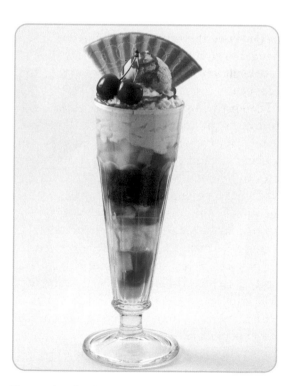

Too much refined sugar in one go can send the body's internal chemistry into overdrive and lead to excess fat deposits

Caffeine

This is a stimulant that is not just found in coffee but also in tea at lower levels, as well as in many cola or fizzy drinks and over-the-counter medicines. Caffeine can become addictive, meaning that over time the body builds up a tolerance to it so higher levels are required to achieve the same effect. It can produce tremors or shaking limbs if used in extremely high doses – for example, drinking more than 6 cups of strong, fresh-brewed coffee per day. If you are used to high levels of caffeine, reducing your intake can have side effects such as headaches, irritability and tiredness. Caffeine stimulates your adrenal glands, which sit over your kidneys, to produce a hormone called adrenalin, which is linked to the 'fight or flight' response. This hormone increases your blood pressure and sends energy to your muscles; useful if you

need to run, but if it is not used up it can have a depleting effect on the body, causing tiredness and also decreasing the effectiveness of the immune system. If you monitor your intake of caffeine for a few days, via tea, coffee or cola drinks, again try to note when you take it, why, and *how you feel* when you think you 'need it'. If you find you are reaching for caffeine every time you feel mentally tired or depleted, this is a signal that your body really needs proper rest so you can clearly assess what is happening to you.

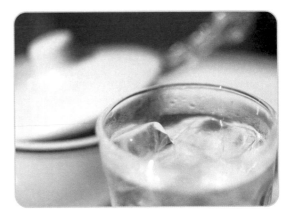

Drinking several glasses of pure spring water each day is a simple way to cleanse and detoxify your system

A note about water

Caffeine and sugar together, for example in cola-type drinks, are a potent combination that lead to more thirst and more drinking, and so on. It is very common these days to find that many people are actually dehydrated, even though they think they are drinking plenty of liquid. The liver and kidneys have to detoxify and filter all the chemicals out of soft drinks before the fluid can be used. All the body's systems require water and the internal management of stress symptoms themselves can place further burdens on the body's water resources. The body needs *pure* water. We are made up of roughly 80 per cent water in

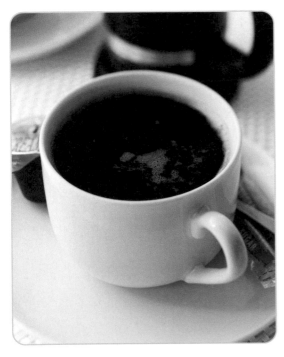

Drinking more than two cups of strong coffee a day can give you tremors and shakes and stop you from sleeping

total – only 20 per cent solids, believe it or not – and we need to replace water daily. One of the simplest and best detoxifying and inner-cleansing tools you can try is to drink eight large glasses of pure spring water daily, as well as reducing your intake of drinks high in caffeine like coffee, tea or cola or, better still, removing them altogether.

Factors with stronger addictive potential

Alcohol

This is a colourless liquid produced by using yeast to ferment carbohydrates found in plants like wheat (to make whisky) or grapes (to make wine) or potatoes (to make vodka). Alcohol is considered to be a drug. It has a swift effect on the brain and central nervous system, initially reducing anxiety, tension and social inhibitions. If levels in the body get higher, then reactions will slow and there can be difficulty staying upright. Extreme levels of alcohol in the system can cause unconsciousness or even breathing difficulties. If high levels of alcohol are consumed over a longer period of time, the body will start to show signs of damage to the brain itself, as well as to the heart, digestive system and the liver, which is the body's major organ of detoxification. Like caffeine, alcohol begins to be tolerated by the body at certain

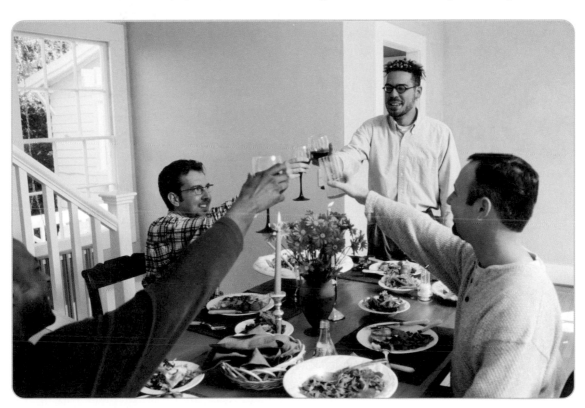

Moderate intake of alcohol, such as a glass or two of wine, is not likely to cause you harm and is a pleasant accompaniment to a meal

levels, so over time more needs to be taken to achieve the same effect. This problem lies at the root of alcohol dependency. The easy availability of alcohol and its involvement in most social interactions makes it a very common lifestyle factor. As we said earlier, the key to its effect lies in how much you feel you need it. If you take a small amount here and there, and it makes no difference to how you feel about whether you have it or not, then enjoy a moderate amount; for example, a glass or two of wine with a meal. If you feel really stressed and 'need a drink' every time you come in from work, that is a sign of an underlying pattern you may need to look at. The need for the alcohol may well be giving a false sense of relief from an issue you have not addressed. There are many ways to get help with alcohol dependency; for example, through organisations like Alcoholics Anonymous, or by seeking the advice of your doctor. However, it is not simply a question of giving up alcohol, the important issue to explore is why you feel you need it.

Smoking

Cigarettes contain at least 16 potential cancer-producing chemicals as well as nicotine, which is an addictive substance considered to be a drug. A high amount of nicotine acts like a tranquilliser, giving a sense of relaxation, but it can also increase the amount of adrenalin in the body so that, over time, many heavy smokers start to suffer from high blood pressure. The effects of nicotine depend on how many cigarettes are smoked and how accustomed a person's system is to the drug. Nicotine can also reduce the appetite, which is why some women say they smoke to keep their weight down; they then wonder why their weight goes up when they give up – perhaps it's because their appetite is back to

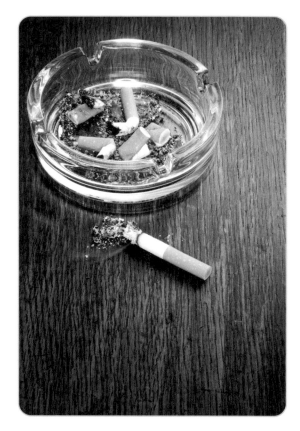

Nicotine, which is found in cigarettes, is a drug which can very easily become addictive. Over time it can cause high blood pressure

normal. Smoking can also cause many other well-known potential harmful effects to the lungs and the heart. Like any habit, it is useful to look at why a person thinks they need it and what 'reward' they think it gives them. There are many social and peer pressures still associated with smoking, especially among young people. Many people smoke to feel relaxed. However, the risks to health over a long period far outweigh any relaxation they might feel, and there are many other ways to achieve a sense of well-being – as we have already seen in other chapters. Giving up smoking, particularly if it has been a habit for some time, can be challenging; as the nicotine is the addictive substance, the use of patches or gum that release it into the bloodstream are fairly successful tools to help combat addiction, as long as they do not become substitutes. It is very useful to get help and support from your doctor if you are serious about giving up smoking.

Drug dependency

This is a complex area and we have already seen examples of some types of drugs – caffeine, alcohol and nicotine. However, the deliberate taking of illegal drugs such as marijuana, cocaine or heroin or so-called 'designer drugs' like Ecstasy is an issue that is affecting more and more sections of the population, including young people. Discussing the long-term effects of such habits is beyond the remit of this book, but the topic deserves to be raised in the context of stress-related symptoms. The need to escape from reality, to feel relief from burdens or problems, to experience a state where pressures disappear and there is a sense of euphoria – these are some reasons why drugs may seem attractive, at least at first. Their addictive effects mean that once a person is 'hooked', the need for those experiences becomes a driving force.

Dependency here requires medical and psychological help at a professional level.

The reason for raising all these lifestyle factors is that they are very present in today's world. Though their symptoms and signs are readily known, they also imply some level of underlying need. As well as understanding the effects of these factors at an addictive level, it is useful in the context of stress management to look closely at why someone requires them. They point to a deep level of physical, mental or emotional pressure. A person may feel they cannot cope unless they use one of these types of prop. If stress levels are pushing a person to this extent, they really would benefit from some professional support. Often, if someone can actually admit that they have an underlying problem, this is a major step towards their own recovery.

casestudy

This is an example of someone with a severe caffeine addiction. Paul was a manager I worked for some years ago. He would drink strong black coffee from the moment he arrived at work to the time he went home. If you were in a meeting with him there were times when his hands would shake, he would be irritable and he would react irrationally. Looking back at his situation, I can see that he was surrounded by younger colleagues at a time when the company was changing structure. He had real concerns about his own future and he used coffee as a way to keep himself alert and on the lookout for anyone who might trip him up. The trouble was, the coffee was having a negative effect on his general health, particularly his digestion and his blood pressure, and he was so used to it he had stopped noticing. After I left the company I heard that his health became worse, and in the end he was retired early on ill-health grounds.

Consider these questions:

1 Can you see the underlying emotion here that was driving Paul along?

2 How do you think that emotion contributed to his poor health?

3 Do you have any ideas about how he might have improved things?

When it comes to lifestyle factors linked to stress, it's important to be honest with yourself. That way you may be able to identify a pattern, notice when it is happening and consider why that might be. To do this takes courage because it might mean you have to admit something to yourself that you have been hiding. For many people that is too daunting and they prefer not to look at the cause. However, the decision to see it has to rest with them. It is ironic that even if someone points your pattern out to you, you may be the best person to hide it from yourself. Life is full of challenges and it is how we meet them that really matters. To make real progress, the willingness to see things as they really are has to be there within you.

FAQs

I admit I like a drink or two most evenings when I come in – it is a habit. I acknowledge that, and I use the alcohol to help me relax. I think I'm entitled to it after working hard. Are you going to tell me I have a problem?

No, it's not up to me to say. As long as you are aware of how much you are drinking and your consumption does not start to creep upwards, it is unlikely to be causing you harm. Just notice that you believe the alcohol is a reward for your hard work. Are there any other ways you could give yourself that reward?

Does it make a difference what kind of coffee you drink – that is, instant versus fresh-ground coffee?

All coffee contains caffeine, but instant coffee is often processed with other chemicals that may be detrimental to health, as well as the caffeine it contains. Freshly ground coffee *in small amounts* is actually likely to do you less damage.

What about decaffeinated coffee?

Caffeine is not the only stimulant in coffee; removing it still leaves two other potential stimulants behind. If you are really keen on a coffee-type taste, try substitutes made with roasted barley or chicory.

What about 'diet' drinks with artificial sweeteners – aren't they better for you than the ones with sugar?

Definitely not – a 'diet' drink is water with a cocktail of artificial chemical tastes, colourings and sweeteners. Sweeteners like aspartame have been linked to physical conditions like headaches or dizziness. They really are best avoided.

Water tastes really boring on its own – I can't make myself drink those big glasses of it. What can I do?

Some people swear by drinking it out of a beautiful glass! Otherwise, you can carry a bottle of water with you and drink it steadily throughout the day. This is especially good to do during the summer months. It's surprising how much you will drink if you take your water gradually and it can help your body to absorb it better.

I know someone who gave up smoking 'just like that' after years of a heavy habit. How was that possible?

Success in giving up smoking does depend a great deal on the individual. Some people find it is very hard, and others seem to be able to stop, as you say, 'just like that'. This may be due to compelling health reasons, or possibly because someone has just decided they do not need cigarettes any more. The power of the mind can be very significant in this.

How do you really know when one of these lifestyle factors is getting towards an addictive level?

Simply when it gets to the point where you absolutely cannot do without it, or if stopping using it would be a real problem for you. If the craving or desire for the reward is overwhelming, that may be a sign of a pattern you should look at.

more stress-beating strategies

Looking back over our journey, in Section 1 of this book we examined stress and how it occurs, and in Section 2 we explored ways to deal with physical, mental and emotional stress patterns, as well as recognising important lifestyle factors. Here in Section 3, we are going to work with some key stress-beating strategies that go straight to core areas of your life where stress may start to manifest. Get these areas of your life sorted out and you will be much better prepared to deal with potential stressors as they occur. First, we will deal with your concept of your own space; then with getting motivated; and finally with the concept of change. Use these chapters to help you launch yourself into a fresh phase of your life!

clearing your personal space

8

What do you understand by your 'personal space'? It can mean many things. It can mean how you feel about yourself on the inside as well as on the outside. It can mean your space on a practical level, like the place where you live or the car you drive, for example. In this chapter you will begin to see that your 'personal space' extends into many aspects of your life that you can see and touch, and these levels contain real clues about your stress levels. Why? Because the way you behave or react will always show up in the area of your personal space. If you open your eyes you will find all sorts of information about what is going on in your life right there in front of you. The good news is, if you are prepared to roll up your sleeves and actually do some work, and this may actually mean some physical effort, you can literally clear your personal space and get some 'room to breathe'. If your personal space is full of 'stuff', you will never be able to think clearly or make useful decisions. The great thing about exploring your 'personal space' is that you can see really quickly how to make changes, and as soon as you make them you feel the benefits.

Stress and personal space

Stress levels affect your 'personal space' in many ways and if you look closely you will begin to see the clues. When you are stressed, for whatever reason, it affects the choices you make and the things you decide to do – or not to do. This immediately has an effect on your surroundings. If you let the pattern go on for a long time, you may very well end up feeling overwhelmed. This is why there is a fashion for TV programmes where people let their houses be cleared by somebody else. In one show, a woman lived in a small house and she had so much 'stuff' that when it was all laid out in the back garden the pile was higher than her house . . . and it had all been *in* there before! Her need to surround herself like this stemmed from huge emotional insecurity, and initially she found her emptier space to be quite challenging. However, she managed to resist the impulse to fill it up again, and in so doing lost weight, gained a better social life and made a new start. This is a very real example of the power of personal space.

In Japan and other eastern countries, there is respect for personal space and an attention to creating as clear an area as possible for living, being, breathing and meditating. Temples are cleansed and fragranced daily, but so are homes and personal shrines. Even if spaces are small, if they are clear then they can reflect a feeling of peace and openness, and a simple bowl of fresh flowers or a lit candle transmits a feeling of tranquillity and balance. This is what happens when personal space is worked with using focus and intent, so clearing the outside aspect – what you see and live in – creates room for the inner aspect – your inner feelings – to develop and grow.

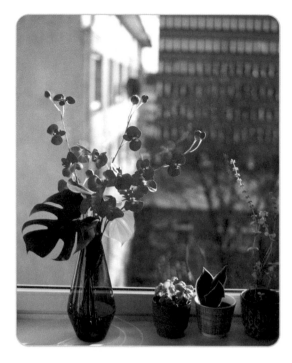

In the East, spaces are cleansed and kept free of clutter to help calm the mind as well as create an open area

Letting go

In the West we have grown very used to filling our spaces to the absolute brim to demonstrate our buying success, the power of our purses, or the level of our credit cards. This is all very well, but it can create an obsession with things leading to more things and more things still, until it just gets too much. When did you last move house? Why was it so overwhelming? What does everybody say – 'Isn't it amazing how much stuff you accumulate?' It's ironic that so many people create more and more financial stress for themselves by buying bigger houses to fit all their things into because they 'need more room'. If you really boil it down, we need very

little to survive. We have just decided to want a lot more. It's a question of choice . . . and of course, the global economy relies on us continuing to want more . . . but does this really make us happy? Think about that question and answer it honestly for yourself. What about Christmas, which has become the most ridiculously commercialised excuse for consumerism, far removed from the original spirit of a festival designed to give thanks for new light. Listen to people in supermarket queues – 'I don't know how we are going to afford it all this year . . .' There is a stress level showing up. Christmas is a great time for accumulation.

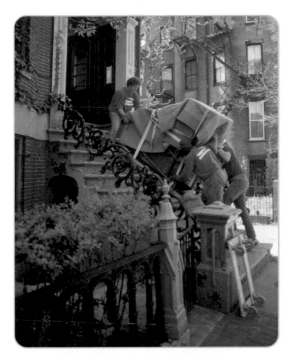

Moving house can be made even more stressful if you have accumulated a lot of things and you need more space to put them in

things can be painful. Yet the release creates a sense of lightness and openness, both physically and emotionally. In an open, spacious environment your body, mind and emotions can relax much more easily, and stress levels decrease.

To start experiencing what this is all about, we will be looking at ways to work at what is called space clearing. This is an aspect of a much wider art from the East called 'Feng Shui', which starts with clearing so that objects that are necessary can then be placed carefully in the most energising locations. You can find out about the art of placement via many books on Feng Shui, and its full practice is beyond our remit here. However, space clearing is a technique from that tradition which is easy to try and very useful to us. We will work with it in two key areas: your house, which is the main one, and your car. We will then apply some of its principles to you, looking at how you treat yourself. Space clearing can be done alone, but it does help on a practical level to have someone else with you, like a friend or relative. The reason for this is that sometimes you may need a bit of persuasion to let go of some things . . .

Is it possible to reverse this trend? Yes it is, but it can takes some mental discipline and a lot of emotional understanding. Letting go of

Clearing your home

If you've decided to clear your home space, congratulations – that is a real step forward! Now be reassured we are not going to take you back to bare floorboards and packing cases. We are simply going to go through what is in your space in a steady, methodical way and let you decide what you really want to keep and what you can release.

Before you start in depth, a simple preparation is to go through the main living areas and clear away any obvious surface clutter, like old newspapers, magazines,

telephone directories, all those items of 'junk mail' that accumulate so easily and any other obvious rubbish. Then decide on one area of your home where you would like to begin. Rather than going at this in a haphazard way, see it through, notice how that makes you feel and then go on to another area. It really pays to be methodical.

Go through the space looking at all the things it contains. Ask yourself – and answer honestly – 'Do I really need this NOW?' You may have needed some things at some point

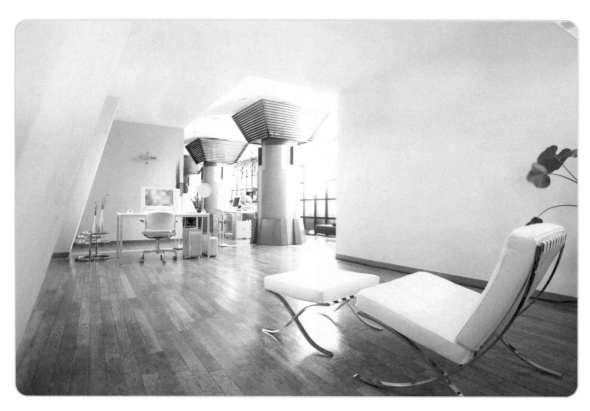

Clear open space is relaxing and soothing to mind and body, and becomes a real sanctuary

in the past but they may not be relevant any more. Check each item and consider whether it is still important to you. If you want to keep something, be clear why; there may be practical or emotional reasons for choosing to let it stay, but be clear what these are. This is why it's good to have a friend with you because you can talk this through as you go along. What tends to happen is that you start this process slowly, and it feels quite daunting to begin with, and then suddenly a momentum builds and it gets faster. You just know what is to go and what is to stay, and you experience a sudden burst of energy as you start to feel the space opening up.

When you have ended up with a pile of things to go, consider how you will dispose of them – old books and knick-knacks to charity shops, for example, and electrical items that no longer work to the local waste disposal site. Deal with the fallout from one area at a time, so you can decide what is going and complete the process of releasing before you move on to the next area. This is a real psychological boost. Notice how you feel in the area you have cleared. What is its quality now? You may want to give it a really good spring clean or a new coat of paint, to burn some incense to cleanse the air or to put some fresh flowers in a lovely vase to bring in colours. This is a great way to begin.

People who have the courage – and it takes courage – to clear their entire space can feel very powerful effects. One woman I know took it on having forgotten that a lot of her father's things had been sitting in her garage since his death, so not only did she clear her belongings but his too, which she had been keeping in her space. Deciding to keep a few important personal items of his and letting go of the rest was a significant stage in her life's journey. Some people who let go of a lot of accumulation on the physical level find that their weight decreases too. It's probably because their whole life suddenly got lighter.

The only way to find out how this process will affect you is to try it, so here is a challenge. Go into your space and choose one small area, – a desk, for example. Spend some time really clearing the clutter and sorting out what you need to keep. Notice how much you end up throwing away. When you have finished, make a simple gesture to show that the space is now clear; lighting one simple candle in it is an easy technique to use. Notice how it feels to be in the space now. Which do you prefer – how it was before, or how it is now? I hope you will be inspired to take this approach right through your home. If you do, the feeling you receive from the peaceful open space outside you will

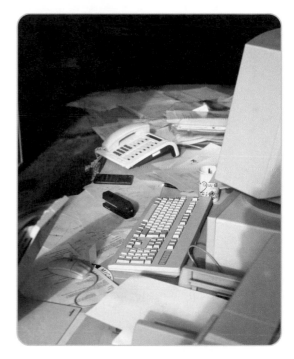

Starting with one small area and really going through it carefully is a simple and effective way to see the benefits of space clearing

reach deep inside you. No matter what happens to you during daily life, if your home space is clear, you can be clear. It can become a sanctuary for you, a true place of rest and release from pressure and tension.

Clearing your car

Obviously not everyone has a car, but if you do you may like to take a look at it in the light of the previous exercise. Often the level of clutter in the house is mirrored in the car, which is the means whereby you transport yourself through your world. Many people feel that their car is an extension of their home space and they

relate to it in a similar way; notice car manu-facturers are creating and adding extra features like DVD and game-playing equipment to rear seats, which make the car more and more like the living room at home. If you have a car, go and take a look at it. Look at its external state, how clean it is on the outside, and think about how well you maintain it. It does a valuable job for you by taking you where you need to go and it also says something about how you move through your world. Do you want to move around in a messy state or in a clear and open state? Clean the car, clean the windows, let some light in. Have a look inside and get rid of all the rubbish – the old parking tickets and sweet wrappers. Clean out the interior properly. When it's done, take it for a drive and see how it feels now. It may seem like a small thing, but it is another level of help you are giving yourself in part of your personal environment. If it feels good to be in the car then the stress of driving may be slightly diminished!

Clearing yourself

I'm not suggesting you take a brush and scrub yourself with bathroom cleaner! However, if the principles of space clearing apply to your external space, then why not to you too? By this I mean thinking about looking after yourself. The media places enormous emphasis on physical appearance but this is not what I'm getting at. I'm talking about how you treat yourself. When people are under severe stress they tend to stop taking care of themselves. This can be difficult to identify just by looking at someone, as today's fashion trends seem to maximise the messy and 'just-out-of-bed' look. However there are still signs and the reason why TV make-over shows are so popular is because they take people who have forgotten how to look after their appearance and try to turn them around. A woman on a recent show put up a physical struggle when she was separated from the shapeless baggy tracksuit trousers she wore every day. However, there is a deeper level at work when someone is not taking care of themselves. It is not just about external appearance, it is also about how they feel inside. It may be that they don't feel worthy or able to give themselves that level of care. However, if this is how *you* feel, take a risk and allow yourself to choose differently. Allow yourself to think yes, I really deserve to receive something good for me . . . and make it happen!

Starting to take care of yourself again can be fun. Take yourself out for an invigorating walk somewhere, or get yourself a massage or a special treatment, or perhaps invest in a fitness programme as a real commitment to a new phase in your life. Make a point at least once a week of doing something just for you that really contributes to your relaxation, health and well-being; the psychological boost is very significant. It creates a more enhanced sense of your inner self. This, plus an enhanced sense of your home as a sanctuary, is a real platform for positive change. As they say – watch this space!

Notice how in the following case study, in the example of the retreat centre startled Barry into realising how cluttered his own space was.

casestudy

A friend of mine called Barry went through a very difficult period in his life when his partner left him and he found it really hard to keep everything together in his job. He ended up being signed off sick for stress-related anxiety. This went on for a few months. During that time he was inspired to take himself away on a meditation retreat to a Buddhist centre in the countryside, here in the UK. The simplicity of the retreat centre and the living space there really impressed him and he found great benefit in experiencing meditation in the external peace of that environment. He noticed it had a knock-on effect by helping him to feel more balanced on the inside. When he came home he saw how his home space was the exact opposite of the place he had visited – it was dirty, cluttered and untidy. He applied himself to a clearing process with real commitment and continued his mediation practice in his own space once it was prepared. He is now in a totally different personal space and life is moving forward positively for him.

Consider these questions:

1 Think about your own living space at this moment. How relaxing and supportive is it for you to be in?

2 Can you see how you might change this for the better?

FAQs

How can you do this space clearing if you live in a space shared with others?

It's possibly more complex to set up but it can become a point of focus and beneficial change if everyone can agree to be involved in the process. As we said earlier, start with one shared space, like a living room, and see how people feel when the clutter is removed and there is a more open atmosphere.

I am embarrassed to say I have so much stuff in my little flat I would be ashamed to show it to anyone – but I can't get started on clearing it either because it seems like too big a job for me. Help!

This is a situation where getting a really sympathetic friend involved is a good idea. Remember, they are there to help not to judge you, and because they are impartial they can help you make choices when it feels tough. Don't take on too much too soon; set out to achieve some progress in a specific area and notice how you feel when that is done.

What if you throw something away and then regret it later?

That is just tough, I'm afraid, and it does point to the need to consider things carefully before you decide what to do with them.

Aren't you just passing on clutter to someone else?

Not if you donate clothes and household items to collections for the needy. You may get notices through your letter box asking for items for people in poorer countries, and this way you pass on things which can be very useful to others.

Is it a good idea to include your wardrobe in the clearing?

Absolutely! This is a whole area in itself, of course, because your clothes really reflect who you are. A common rule of thumb is – if you haven't worn something for a year, are you likely to wear it again? Also, get rid of items that are worn out or shapeless Better still, clear out the new things (usually impulse buys) that have never seen the light of day.

I can't get my head around this idea of giving yourself treats – isn't that just compensating again?

If you look back, the kind of suggestions that were made in this context were things like massage, treatments or fitness sessions that make you feel good about yourself. The idea is that you should use this time to take better care of yourself.

building
self-esteem

9

We human beings are complex, emotional creatures. Our sensitive feelings are easily attacked by stress patterns that can affect our self-esteem (how much we actually like ourselves). Emotional or mental pressures in particular are very good at invading core areas of our inner self-image, eating away at feelings of well-being and contributing to lower levels of self-liking and acceptance. We're all affected in this way at some time or other, for different reasons. Sometimes we can rebuild our self-esteem ourselves, or with support from others. However, persistent stress patterns that keep on reinforcing our low self-esteem can make us think 'Well, I really must be like this', and we end up believing it. If this way of thinking carries on unchallenged, we are setting ourselves up for a continuous stress-fuelled loop of low self-approval.

Is that really how we want to live our lives? Is that what we were created for? Think about the miracle of childbirth, which happens every day. Think about the complex set of circumstances and the nine months' preparation in your mother's womb that paved the way for you to be here, now, living your life. Is this what it was all for? Were we just put here to scurry around like mice in a cage, imprisoned by levels of limited and self-critical beliefs?

In this chapter we are going to take a look at self-esteem, how much we like ourselves, and find out ways to help rebuild our inner sense of self-worth. Let's start from a point that says we all have something to dislike or criticise about ourselves – we are all equal here. If you are working in a group answering the questions that come up later in the chapter, remember that sharing the results in pairs or in small groups should be done in an atmosphere of respect and support, and nobody has to disclose anything they are not comfortable with. Any deeper issues may need to be raised with your tutor. If you are working alone and you feel you need more guidance, it may be appropriate to work with a professional counsellor for support.

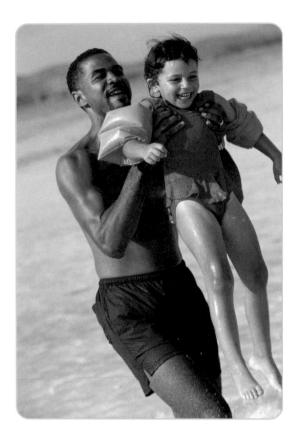

Your early feelings of self-approval were very influenced by the reactions of those around you

However, the questions are meant to bring up key information without going in too deep, and if you can approach them in a space of honesty and clarity you will reap the benefits.

The aim here is to get you started on a new phase in your life where you observe events as they occur and notice if they trigger a reaction that hits your self-esteem. If you feel something *is* hitting you, using the questions here can help you to explore why that might be. You will be able to examine the situation differently so that you can do something about it. This is empowering, and it starts to change the way emotional and mental stress events affect you. You will need your notebook to answer the questions, so have it ready.

The origins of low self-esteem

First, we are going to look at where any feelings of low self-esteem may come from originally. As human beings we are on a learning curve from the moment we are born. We start to relate to our environment as soon as we draw breath, and as we grow, our reactions are constantly coloured by what happens to us. In early childhood we are especially impressionable because we are not yet ready or self-aware enough to make our own decisions. We depend a lot on the opinions of others to build up pictures of how we see ourselves. If we have had encouragement and support, then we are fortunate. However, for various reasons, we may have encountered opinions and feedback which knocked our self-confidence and left us feeling unworthy. These early patterns can be very much influenced by mental or emotional stress and may have built themselves into the fabric of how we see ourselves as adults.

Consider these questions:

Here are some key questions to help you explore your own levels of self-esteem. Read the explanations that follow before answering the questions by writing notes for yourself.

1 If you think of a scale of 1–10, where 1 is virtually non-existent, between 4 and 7 is reasonable and 10 is absolutely amazing, where do you rate your self-esteem right now? Select a number.

Scales like this help you to identify the intensity of a feeling. This is a quick way of showing yourself how far something affects you; remember it as a technique and apply it in the moment when events come up.

2 If your rating is less than 10, start to think why this might be?

Believe it or not, it is possible to like yourself very much. This is not being big-headed or egotistical; it means you are living your life in a state of self-encouragement and approval. Think about how you encourage your friends or family or people around you. Is it difficult to think of giving that support to yourself? Some people can, and they live very creative lives as a result. If you have a rating of less than 10 write down 2 reasons why you think this might be.

3 What kind of feelings stop you from liking yourself?

Some of these may well be surfacing already. Don't get caught up in them, just be gentle with yourself and observe them. How would you describe these feelings? They could be things like self-doubt, not feeling worthy, shyness, fear or self criticism.

4 In what ways do people show you they appreciate you?

OK, let's turn the situation around for a moment, and think about an occasion where people did give you wonderful feedback and showed you they appreciated you. Write down when it was, what was happening, who was involved and how you felt appreciated. For example, Sally is a member of a choir and never really pushed herself forward to help out with the organisation because she felt shy and unsure whether she could really contribute. On the night of one concert the person in charge of taking the money fell ill and Sally stepped in. She received many thanks from the rest of the admin team and also from the conductor, who acknowledged her personally. She then decided to volunteer to be more involved in the running of things and now she really enjoys this role. Sally felt encouraged to make the change because she acted and received acknowledgement.

5 Do you hold yourself back in life because you don't believe in yourself?

This is a very common situation where an opportunity presents itself and you don't take that step forward because your feelings of self-esteem are low and you don't believe you can. Have a think about the last time this happened to you. What was going on? What kind of opportunity was it? Had similar opportunities come up before and you resisted them? Repetitive situations like this are real pointers to low self-esteem, and the good news is that if you can identify a pattern you can start to change it.

6 Do you put up with things rather than say how you really feel?

This is a common sign of low self-esteem and it may well have its roots in childhood. If you think back, how were your thoughts and opinions received by your family members or your teachers? If this was a positive experience for you then your levels of self-approval are likely to be higher; if you were discouraged from expressing your thoughts or feelings or had negative feedback, especially if this happened regularly, then you may have become used to keeping your thoughts to yourself – because it felt easier or safer. However, *the inner resentment that builds up through this pattern can become powerful over time.*

When you have answers to these six questions, sit and read them through and notice any situations or feelings that repeat themselves, or people who appear regularly in your mind. Make any further relevant notes before moving on.

Forgiveness visualisation

This is a technique you can use directed towards either a situation or a person who you have identified as a source of your low self-esteem. Sit quietly in a comfortable chair, take a few deep breaths and close your eyes. Now visualize a plain white screen in front of your eyes. As you look at the screen, see a picture forming. It can be of the situation you have identified, in which case you see the place, the time and the people involved, or it can be a particular person you have identified as a source of negative feedback to you. Let the image form completely. Replay the feelings you felt – the way events happened, or

how it was to deal with the person concerned – but only for a few moments. Now breathe deeply and address the image, either aloud or in your mind. Say to it, 'I acknowledge that what was said or done happened at that time. Maybe there were other circumstances happening that I could not see. I now forgive the people or the circumstances or the person involved, and let the feelings I have carried just dissolve in golden light.'

Practise this visualisation regularly; you may find if you have identified a persistent pattern you may need to do it more than once. It is a useful technique to help dissolve old beliefs.

Spring-cleaning guilt

Following on from our last chapter, which was about space clearing, there is a level of inner cleansing that can be very useful to dissolve issues around guilt. Guilty feelings can really hold you back from new experiences, and are often triggered by stress-fired reactions in difficult situations. The trouble with guilt is that it tends to hang around, so it can continue to influence how you react over a long period of time. Guilt can also relate back to events that happened a long time ago, and it may contribute to stress levels

if the feelings have not been resolved. Here are some simple steps showing how to take a look at feelings of guilt and how to move through them.

1 Go back over your memory of the event and check what really happened.

Even if the situation happened a long time ago, be clear about all the things you can remember, and if there are other people involved, it may be useful to talk to them to see what they remember. The purpose of this is to try to understand exactly what happened in the situation.

2 Take steps to try, if you can, to achieve some kind of resolution.

You can't change what happened; that event is over. You *can* change how you react to it now. You may find a new level of understanding around why it happened. Even if the outcome makes it impossible for you to communicate directly with the person or people concerned, you can change how you feel about the situation within yourself. Sometimes writing your feelings down in detail is useful. Try burning the paper afterwards and letting the energy of fire cleanse away the feelings.

3 Make a practical gesture to show you are moving on.

This is as much for you as for the other party involved in the situation. Here is an example. Jean and Chrissie were best friends for over ten years – almost like sisters. Chrissie was always in trouble with her relationships and Jean was always there to help her. Then they fell out over a time when Jean needed support but, due to a combination of personal circumstances, Chrissie could not give it to her. They were out of touch for a long time. Jean felt very bitter and Chrissie felt guilty over the lack of communication, but she could never pluck up the courage to pick up the phone. Then one day Chrissie and Jean literally bumped into each other. They were really surprised. It was not easy to talk to each other and it felt awkward. Chrissie wanted to explain why she had not been able to be there for Jean, but the old closeness had gone. She came home, wrote down her reasons – which had been genuine – and all her feelings. She burned the paper

afterwards, and buried the ashes in her garden. Then she planted a rose bush in the spot as a symbol of new growth. She wanted to move on from the feelings and, although she could not achieve actual resolution with Jean, she found that this process meant she could move on and not feel guilt anymore.

Understanding how feelings of low self-esteem have come about and cleansing away any remaining guilt levels is a beneficial way to begin rebuilding feelings of self-approval. Here is another exercise to try. How would life be different if you really believed in yourself? If you could act, think, speak and react from a place inside you that believes you deserve the very best, how might your circumstances look? Create your own screenplay of unfolding events that reflect you in a position of confidence and self-belief. Take one aspect of your life, such as your work, and think about it like this. See if you can describe how you might be, and most important, FEEL the difference inside you when you put yourself in this situation. That feeling can become real if you open up to it.

Here is another example. Sandra has worked hard all her life but has been stopped from really progressing in her job because she does not have a university degree. She has always believed that she was not intelligent enough to do a degree, and now that she is 43 she also feels she is too old to start. She does not have very high level school qualifications and although she has done some training through work, for example in computer skills, she does not see herself as academically capable. Then Sandra decides to get some advice about her career prospects and the idea of a degree comes up again. Using the questions in this chapter, Sandra realises that as a child she grew up in a family where education was not really valued and earning money was more important. If she was caught reading books, she was told off for doing nothing. Over time she put up with this and accepted it rather than get into conflict. Now she sees how this pattern has really held her back. She has also forgiven her parents for their influence on her life, realizing that they were only reflecting their level of understanding at the time. She has taken on an access course to get qualified at the right level and is now doing a degree in management studies on a part-time basis. She feels her attitudes are changing towards success and her future prospects are now greatly improved.

Identifying areas where your self-esteem is low, working to understand why this has happened and clearing old patterns will help you to create a fresh feeling of optimism in your life. Stressful events will still occur, but if you are reacting to them from a place inside you that knows your own worth, these stresses will not bite so deeply. You will feel much more able to make choices that serve you and improve your life experience.

FAQs

My self-esteem is around 6 on the scale – somewhere in the middle. Isn't that normal?

It depends what you mean by normal – the value may not be normal to someone else. If by this you mean that your self-esteem will tend to float around that middle area and never go up or down a great deal, perhaps you may like to consider what that may be saying about you and your life at the moment.

Isn't it being big-headed to 'like yourself'?

Why? This question shows there is an embedded attitude that is still very prevalent, saying that self-approval is wrong or selfish or egotistical. This is simply not true. To approve of yourself and to like who you are is a healthy state of being that allows you to react positively to events in your life.

Sometimes you have to take knocks in life and just get on with it. Surely you can't always wait for somebody else to pat you on the head in approval?

Considering how other people appreciate you is not the same as waiting for pats on the head. It means noticing what kind of situations generate that kind of spontaneous reaction from people, and then how that makes you feel. We tend to be very good at recalling when we are criticised, and less aware of when we are praised. That is the pattern we are trying to reverse.

You simply can't always expect life to go the way you want – sometimes you have to put up and shut up. Surely that is realistic?

No, I would say that to put up and shut up is a always choice you make in the moment. It may not feel that is the case because it is something you have become really used to doing. It's a reaction that becomes deeply ingrained over time, and therefore difficult to shift. If you are finding this happens a lot in your life, I would suggest you take some time to find out why.

Isn't imagining yourself in a better situation just 'pie in the sky'?

Creative visualisation, where you 'see yourself' in a situation that is more positive, is a real tool for change. It allows you to 'feel' what that situation might be like if it had a positive charge. This can then encourage you to experiment with your reactions in real time and enable you to make new choices.

I'm 46 and my mother still criticises my hair and my appearance! Can you believe that? It still gets to me and I feel like a child. What can I do?

I think this may need some work with the forgiveness visualisation, especially if you can't achieve any resolution with your mother face to face. Perhaps if you take time to consider why she feels the need to keep on criticising you, you may discover something about her. If you can use the visualisation to simply forgive her for her need to do this, then her behaviour may at least stop affecting you. There is a hint of bullying here, and bullies tend to lose interest if their behaviour doesn't cause a reaction.

coping with change

When you talk to people about how they perceive stress, these days it's very common to hear phrases like 'Everything moves so fast' or 'I just can't keep up with it all' or 'I think time is speeding up.' Sometimes you might hear comments like 'Why can't things stay the same?', 'It wasn't like this in my day' or 'You just can't take anything for granted any more.' All of these expressions show a reaction to change. Change is always present in the fast-paced lives we live and manifests itself in many ways. Only a few generations ago the expectancy was that a job was for life and then you retired. Now, you face several potential job changes in a lifetime and that is considered normal. Change is one of the deepest potential stressors at work in our lives today. It can generate anxiety, fear, worry about the future, unsteadiness and feelings of being out of control. Yet the paradox with change is the more you resist it, the more painfully it will affect you. The more you expect events, people or relationships to stay the same or the more you try to hold on to them, the more they seem to slip through your fingers.

The reason for this is simple – change means things will not stay the same. For many people that is a real challenge, which is why

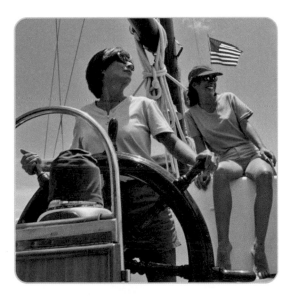

Learn to be the navigator of your own life, so you ride the waves of change with ease

95

change knocks them off balance. If you can turn your perception around and start from a point of view that accepts that change is the norm, that it is the only reality, and work with it instead of against it, then you can be the navigator of your life instead of feeling as though you are at sea in a storm-tossed ship. Then you will allow events to run through your life and give yourself the freedom to choose what is important to you, letting go of what does not serve you and moving on. This way of being is like flowing with a current instead of damming it up.

Maybe that sounds challenging to you; how can you stay grounded if everything is constantly moving? Eastern disciplines like Tai Chi promote the way to find stillness within motion, teaching that finding a centre within yourself which you can breathe into and go back to at any time is the way to stay focussed and aware within the currents of daily life. In Chapter 5 we looked at breathing, meditation, visualisation and simple yoga techniques, which also stem from Eastern traditions. These teachings show that the power to manage change lies within YOU, in that calm centre, a point of stillness. Nobody else can 'make change better' or sort it out for you. You are the navigator of your life, and if you want to manage change and the stress it can cause, then this chapter will give you some suggestions you can use to experiment and feel more comfortable with it.

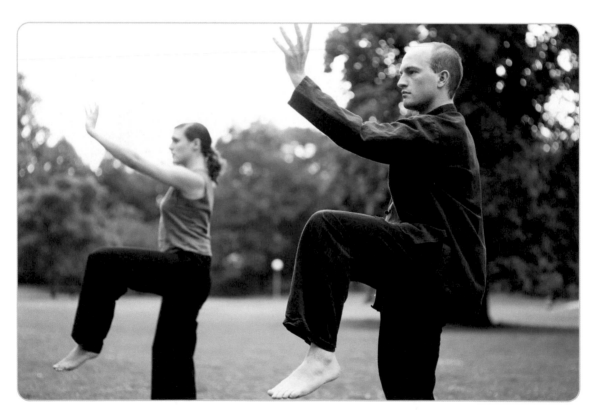

Disciplines like Tai Chi help you to find a point of inner stillness even while you are moving, which is a great help when coping with change

Learning to be in the present

Coping with change is the most transformational of all stress management techniques. Change lies at the very root of life. We are all changing, growing in age and maturity, despite all the efforts of the media and popular culture to try to hold back time. Coping with change means moving beyond a concept of time as a line of events. It means learning to be in the present moment, fully aware of what is around you, and realizing that every instant holds a magical potential for transformation. If you can reach this awareness then life becomes filled with fun, opportunities and possibilities.

Focussing exercise

Let's start with an exercise designed to bring you into focus in this present moment. Sit comfortably with your hands resting in your lap and your feet uncrossed. Take a few deep breaths and feel your body being supported by the chair.

Place your right hand over the middle of your chest and rest the left one on top of it. Sit quietly and breathe regularly, creating an even rhythm. Feel your hands in the centre of your chest, and the gathering warmth underneath them. Let this feeling of warmth and comfort permeate throughout your body as you sit. If any thoughts come up, just let them dissolve. After a few more moments take your hands away and let them sit loosely in your lap. Notice how you feel now, in this moment.

This simple exercise can be used at any time, especially when you need to feel centred. We spend a lot of time out of the present moment by chewing over things that have happened in the past or worrying about the future, which is unknown. If you really think about it, you will realise that the only moment we ever really know fully is the present. The past is the past, it's gone and finished with, and the future is a realm of possibilities we don't know about yet. The only moment where we are truly alive is the present. If we can start to work from this moment, we begin to realise that this is always the point of change, the place where movement and transformation are possible. If we can bring ourselves into the present then we can make choices in this point of dynamic change.

Learning to be in present time takes practice. Some people do it easily, but for most of us it is a skill we have to relearn. We knew how to be in this place when we were children. If you recall, in childhood the way time worked seemed to be very different – somehow longer, more spacious. It's only

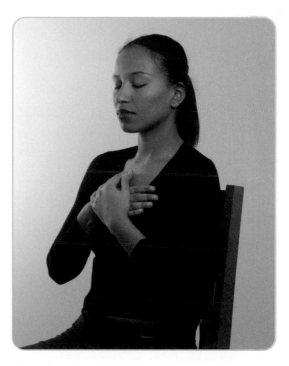

Sit quietly and breathe, enjoying the warmth that spreads from under your hands bringing a sense of peace

when the demands of adult life turn up that time becomes limiting, a thing to be twisted and pushed into the boxes on the calendar, a commodity that becomes scarce. 'I wish I had more time.' How often do you hear that? Learning to be in the present moment is fascinating because it actually seems to expand time once again. It is a vital muscle to build up to enable you to cope better with change.

Let's explore two types of exercises to get you playing with the present moment. A spirit of play is very important because it brings in fun and spontaneity, which are vital elements of present experience. In the first set of exercises you are invited to choose to change something you do all the time in a small way, to see how that feels. In the second set, you are invited to be spontaneous and see what happens!

Experimenting with change

These exercises can be done as homework tasks or, if you are working on your own, you could try one at a time and see how you get on. It's important to observe your feelings closely when you try an exercise because these are key

pointers to how you react to change. The list contains some suggestions, so if you can think of other ideas you would like to experiment with, by all means try them out!

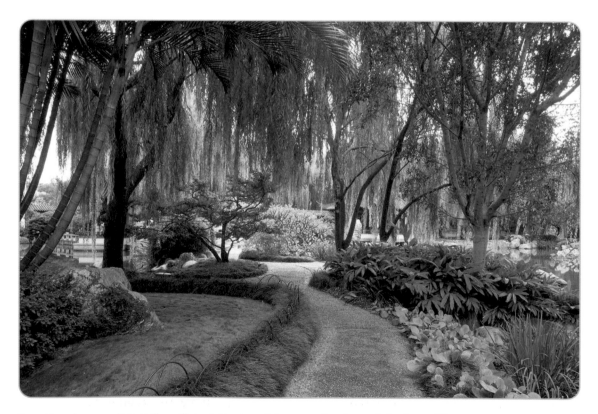

Even if you know a place really well, try taking a walk in a new direction or following a different route

A new walk

Visit a park or another location you know well. Go for a walk, but take a totally different route to the one you normally follow. Take new turnings as often as you can. If you see a direction you want to follow then do so. Choose to change paths as often as possible. See what unfolds. How do you perceive this space now? What do you see? Anything new? How does that feel?

A new journey to work

Most of us take the same routine journey to work each day – week in, week out. There are always other options to try. Just for a few days, make an effort to travel to work along a different route. Get off the bus and walk a bit, or use your bicycle. If you are driving, choose a different route and try it out – you never know, it might turn out to be quicker or more pleasant. Notice the effect that seeing a different part of town has on your thoughts.

A different mode of transport

This can be great fun. In many cities there are different ways to travel; for example, in London there is a thriving riverboat service that stops at different points. Investigate your local area, see what is on offer, and try out a

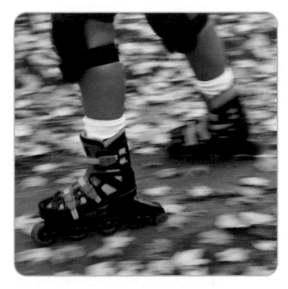

Try out a different type of transport and you may even get fitter into the bargain

different way of getting from A to B. Notice how that feels.

A new colour

What we choose to wear can become very much a habit, particularly in an office environment. For a change, try wearing a colour you would not normally choose. You could try a scarf or a tie in a more vibrant shade if you don't want to be too obvious. It's amazing what a difference a splash of colour makes to how you feel, and you will be surprised how people notice it!

Exercises for spontaneity

Being spontaneous is a wonderful way to experiment in the present moment and experience change. It's a state of mind we enjoy a lot when we are children but it tends to become buried under the demands of daily adult life. Exercise your spontaneity and you will see things start to happen; it's an energy that releases new events. It brings freshness and a sense of being carefree, which are positive aspects of change.

Here are some suggestions to try, but a word of advice: being spontaneous does not mean booking them into your diary, but rather waking up one day and thinking 'I know! I'll do . . . today!' Then see how you feel after you have enjoyed yourself!

Take yourself out for a treat

Decide on inpulse to do something wonderful for yourself. Here are some ideas: a ride on a merry-go-round, a visit to a place you have never been, old-fashioned tea with scones and cream, a sauna . . .

Buy yourself flowers

This can be a lovely thing to do to bring colour and fragrance into your space; enjoy choosing them and placing them in your environment.

Listen to a new kind of music

Sound is very powerful and can have a an enormous effect on how you feel. Go and hear a kind of music that is new to you, and do it 'live'. Maybe you have never heard a gospel choir, or African drummers, or live jazz, or a classical opera. Give yourself this experience and notice how it affects you.

Ring someone you haven't spoken to for a year

Be spontaneous – ring someone you have lost touch with and see how they are. There's nothing to lose, and you never know what it might trigger!

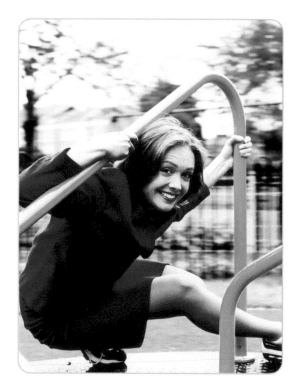

Be spontaneous – do something you have always wanted to do, or something you remember from childhood

These simple experiments with change and spontaneity are designed to be easy and fun to try but they have a real benefit. They start to re-educate you in being in the moment, so you see how life can develop and grow from where you are now. The more you act in the present, the more persistent patterns of boredom or stress just dissolve. Life can get into a rut or into habits that are limiting, and then change seems threatening when it occurs because it upsets what seems like strict order. If you are in the present moment, your life is more fluid and you will find it easier to adapt to unfolding events as they happen.

Another vital tool in the management of change is humour. If you can laugh in the face of adversity, it is amazing how it opens up new ways of seeing things. In Native American teaching, one of the most important animals is the coyote, the wild dog that chases its own tail. It is seen as a symbol of humour, recognising the importance of being able to laugh at the most challenging times and so see your way clear. So often what seems like a crisis can be turned on its head by seeing what is funny about it. Children are great observers of this.

Here's an example that happened recently. My friend Joanne had an absolute disaster with trying to apply hair colour at home and her hair ended up turning green. She was beside herself over this as she had to go out that evening, and she was in a state of total distress. Her seven-year-old son was in the house with two friends and they couldn't understand why

she was upset. 'People have all sorts of hair colours,' said Jack, and he and his friends started laughing. They thought it was really cool! Joanne ended up laughing too, and she calmed right down. She had to go to the hairdresser to sort out the emergency, but the laughter had dissolved her distress.

There is a thread running through here that keeps comes back to being childlike. This does not mean we all have to revert to childhood, but rather that elements of experimentation, spontaneity and humour, which are part of the experience of childhood, make very good tools for dealing with change. We get used to doing things a certain way as adults, and this can be a trap. In the times we live in we have to be flexible, adaptable and visionary. Change is real, it's happening on all levels – in our

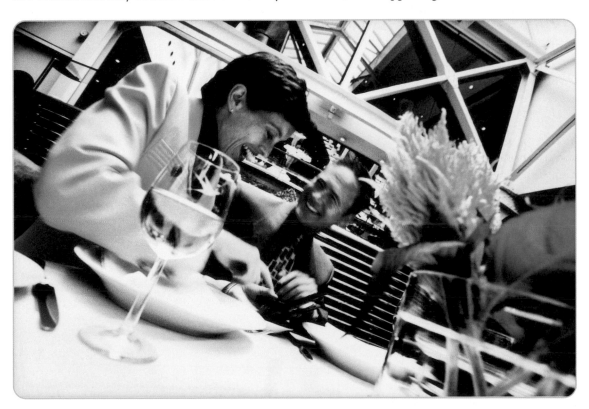

Keeping a sense of humour really helps you to see through changing times and find a new thread to take you forward

bodies, our relationships, the environment, economics, work, politics – even the weather. We can either let this fact create stress levels that make us feel frozen and powerless, or we can exercise our ability to be spontaneous, to play with ideas and to find the humour in situations that will help us get over challenges and move on.

As we said at the beginning of this chapter, change is a fact and if you can accept that it can work *for* you, not *against* you. In terms of managing stress, coping with change is probably the most important skill to learn. The more you practise it, the more you improve, and then life events do not have such a stressful impact. Challenges can turn into opportunities and situations that seem impossible can become filled with potential. Choose to start today and let your life enter a new phase of transformation.

FAQs

I find every time things change I feel thrown off balance. What can I do?

Start to practise a discipline like meditation regularly, every day. The more you do this, the more you will feel centred and calm inside. This centre within you is a key to staying balanced during change.

How can practising Tai Chi or yoga help you cope with change?

These arts teach you how to listen to yourself and find a point of stillness movement, like the eye of a storm. By practising these arts you can become more self-reliant and mentally balanced, so change is not such a threat.

I woke up the other day and wanted to go to the seaside. I actually went and felt so wonderful; it was a magical day. However, when I got back I felt a bit guilty because I had a pile of practical things to do. Why was this?

We are conditioned in this society to think that being spontaneous is not serious or relevant. This is a mistake. Spontaneous decisions can generate a whole new set of ideas and circumstances. I advise you to experiment some more! Incidentally, having fresh levels of energy can get you through the practical things more quickly.

The exercises are all very well, but how do you cope with major changes like losing a job?

The reason for starting simply with the exercises is because, as we said, learning to cope with change is like exercising a muscle. If you start practising now, when major changes come up in life you will have a set of inner practices in place to help you deal with them. Major changes require a deep sense of inner self, a trust in your ability to experiment and a belief in your creativity. Start practising with change and spontaneity now, and be prepared.

I feel a change we simply can't halt is ageing, and that worries me. What can I do?

Learn to appreciate and accept yourself as you are, always. That is the key. We are all changing and we will all age. It is a fact. The media would like us to think otherwise, of course. However the happier you are with yourself on the inside, the more this reflects on the outside. Again, the Eastern disciplines like Tai Chi or yoga are wonderful ways to stay flexible and poised, both inside and outside.

Isn't change exhausting?

It is if you concentrate solely on how it looks on the outside. Then events just make you feel overwhelmed. If you can build your inner awareness you'll observe change from a different perspective and you can choose how you would like to deal with it. There is always a choice, no matter how complex the outside may look.

where to go from here

Coming to the end of this book means you have travelled a long way towards understanding what stress is and how to cope with it in your daily life. If you feel that you would like to go further in your study and exploration of stress patterns and the mind, perhaps to train as a therapist, or if you would like to consult a professional for individual help or guidance, there are different routes you may choose to take.

There are many psychological approaches to choose from and sometimes they do overlap. If you want to consult a therapist, be aware that most therapeutic sessions have to be paid for and very little is available on the NHS. Your doctor is a good point of contact for what the NHS can offer in your area.

Here are some of the main psychological disciplines, briefly outlined.

Counselling

This involves one-to-one sessions with a therapist where specific techniques are used to help a person identify, understand and resolve their issues. There are many different types of counselling approaches but this is a basic definition. Adult education colleges often offer courses in counselling at introductory level and you may even find courses that carry a qualification are available if you decide you would like to practise as a counsellor. If you are looking for a counsellor to consult, then the website for the British Association for Counselling and Psychotherapy is a good point of contact; also for details of courses. The postal address is British Association for Counselling and Psychotherapy, BACP House, 35–37 Albert St, Rugby, Warwickshire, CV21 2SG Tel. 0870 443 5252, *www.bacp.co.uk*. Also consult your doctor to see if counselling is available on the NHS in your area.

Psychotherapy

There are a lot of similarities between counselling and psychotherapy, but perhaps one difference is that in psychotherapy the therapist does not make suggestions, but creates a space for you to find your own answers. Again, this is done through one-to-one sessions. Contact the BACP on the same website, or telephone number, postal address as above for details of registered therapists, if you are looking for professional help, or for courses if you want to study psychotherapy.

Cognitive behavioural therapy

This is an approach that aims to change patterns of behaviour and thinking, using different techniques. It can be offered one-to-one or in group situations. It is helpful for a wide range of problems, including insomnia, anger management and relationship issues. *There is limited availability on the NHS. Check with your doctor for advice.* There is a British Association of Behavioural and Cognitive Psychotherapies, which holds a register of qualified practitioners. Their postal address is BABCP, The Globe Centre, PO Box 9, Accrington BB5 0XB Tel. 01254 875277, *www.babcp.org.uk*

NLP

NLP means neuro-linguistic programming. It is a method of personal development that is designed to improve your performance and can be in any context; for example, in sports or in work. It provides you with models of effective communication, including practical methods to improve how you relate to other people. It also includes the idea of remodelling patterns of human behaviour. NLP can be offered one-to-one or in a group situation. There is a Professional Guild of NLP and their website is *www.nlp-now.co.uk.*

This site contains details of practitioners and available training. The postal address is Pegasus NLP Training, 4 Lyon Close, Yaxley, Suffolk IP23 8BE Tel. 0845 226 0822.

Hypnotherapy

This involves direct interaction, via hypnosis with, a person's inner consciousness. It helps to uncover the root causes of issues in a person's life. Changes of perception at this inner level can be facilitated by the therapist. Hynoptherapy can help you to give up smoking or deal with insomnia or with other deep issues like phobias. If you would like to find a qualified therapist for guidance, the website for the biggest register of hypnotherapy practitioners in the UK is *www.hypnotherapistregister.com* There are many qualifications and associations for hypnotherapy and this website provides the best overview.

Life coaching

This means working one-to-one with a mentor who assists you in identifying and achieving key goals in your life. Sometimes courses in life coaching are offered at beginner level in adult education colleges. To find out more about coaching courses or to find a therapist, the International Coaching Federation has a website, *www.lifecoachingacademy.com.* The postal address is The Coaching Academy UK Ltd, Room 100, Riverbank House, 1 Putney Bridge Approach, London SW6 3JD Tel. 0800 783 4823.

Glossary

Adaptation curve – a graph showing peak levels of stimulation and relaxation related to stress

Addiction – a pattern of behaviour which is repetitive, dominant and dependent on particular circumstances or lifestyle factors

Adrenalin – stimulating stress hormone secreted by the adrenal glands which are situated over the kidneys

Arousal – in stress terms, a peak of stimulation and higher stress

Cognitive behavioural therapy – a combination of techniques bringing together observation of thought patterns and learned behaviour to achieve measurable change

Counselling – one-to-one sessions designed to identify and work through issues

Mantra – from yoga tradition, a sound, which when repeated has a significant effect on brain patterns reducing stress

Meditation – the practice of inner focus to achieve stillness

Psychoanalysis – the analysis of the mind as developed by Freud

Psychology – the study of the mind

Psychotherapy – one-to-one sessions designed to help a client make new decisions around life issues

Space clearing – cleansing clutter to improve the energy in a space

Visualisation – mental images that are used to generate creative thinking

index